Carmen Marie Moniz

THE A-Z OF
WOMEN'S HEALTH

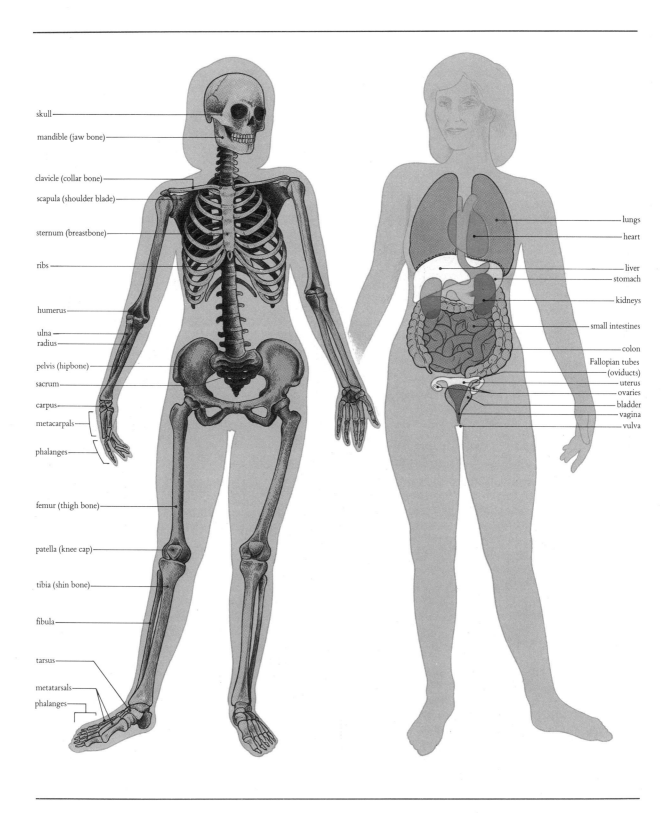

skull

mandible (jaw bone)

clavicle (collar bone)

scapula (shoulder blade)

sternum (breastbone)

ribs

humerus

ulna

radius

pelvis (hipbone)

sacrum

carpus

metacarpals

phalanges

femur (thigh bone)

patella (knee cap)

tibia (shin bone)

fibula

tarsus

metatarsals

phalanges

lungs

heart

liver

stomach

kidneys

small intestines

colon

Fallopian tubes
(oviducts)

uterus

ovaries

bladder

vagina

vulva

The A-Z of WOMEN'S HEALTH

Derek Llewellyn-Jones

OBE, MD, MAO, FRCOG, FRACOG

Oxford University Press/Rainbird
1983

Oxford University Press, Walton Street, Oxford OX2 6DP
London Glasgow New York Toronto
Delhi Bombay Calcutta Madras Karachi
Kuala Lumpur Singapore Hong Kong Tokyo
Nairobi Dar es Salaam Cape Town
Melbourne Wellington
and associates in
Beirut Berlin Ibadan Mexico City Nicosia

First published in 1983 in Great Britain by
Oxford University Press
in association with
The Rainbird Publishing Group Ltd
40 Park Street, London W1Y 4DE
who designed and produced the book

British Library Cataloguing in Publication Data

Llewellyn-Jones, Derek
The A-Z of women's health.
1. Women – Health and hygiene
I. Title
613'.04244   RA778
ISBN 0-19-211589-8

Editors: Georgina Evans & Hilary Dickinson
Designer: Bridget Morley
Artists: Nick Harris; Tony Lodge; Charles Raymond; Ann Savage
Studio services: Radius

Text set by SX Composing Ltd, Rayleigh, Essex, England
Illustrations originated by Bridge Graphics Ltd, Hull, England
Printed and bound by W. S. Cowell Ltd, Ipswich, Suffolk, England

CONTENTS

5

Contents

Preface

In the past two years I have been approached by women, and their partners, who had read my books, *Everywoman, Every Man*, and *Every Body* to ask if I would write a book to complement those books, which they had found to be informative and helpful. The women felt that it would be useful to have an illustrated book, written in the format of a dictionary, available for reference, so that they could obtain a reasonable but concise amount of information about matters concerned with women's health. If they then required further information they would refer to other books – either mine or those of other authors – none of which presents the facts within an immediately accessible alphabetical framework. Armed with this information they would then be able to consult a doctor when necessary – for no book can be a substitute for a doctor, and diagnosis and treatment are dependant upon individual circumstances and the physician's opinion of a patient's total condition.

The concept of an *A-Z of Women's Health* stimulated me, as it meant I would have to rethink the problems and use a different writing technique. This was an agreeable challenge. It was obvious that some selection of topics to be included was required or the book would become too long and too heavy to handle. I was also well aware that certain topics were outside my areas of expertise. For these reasons I have omitted health topics which concern women and men equally or which most commonly affect men, but I have tried to include most health matters which are of concern to women. I am sure that I will have failed to satisfy every reader and would welcome comments and suggestions should sales merit the publication of a new edition.

The list of contents at the front of the book is intended to serve both as a check-list of entries and as an index: information on subjects which do not appear to have their own entry will be found most easily by means of the cross-reference given here. When a subject is mentioned in the text for which there is a separate entry elsewhere in the book, this is shown by an asterisk preceding the appropriate word.

My thanks are especially due to Hilary Dickinson who stimulated me to write the book and who has edited the drafts; to Georgina Evans of Rainbird and Nicholas Wilson of Oxford University Press who have nourished the book from its embryonic stage to its maturity; to Bridget Morley who designed the book; to Carol Kirkland who spent much time typing and retyping the drafts; to Professor Herbert Brant for many useful comments and suggestions at an early stage and Dr Michael Chapman who has helped in checking the copy and artwork.

DEREK LLEWELLYN-JONES
Sydney, Australia, 1983

A

Abortifacients

Folk medicine lists many herbal drugs which, it is claimed, cause abortion or miscarriage. None is effective. Nor are drugs in the medical pharmocopoeia any more effective unless taken in doses which are potentially lethal. Home remedies such as large doses of caster oil, gin by the bottle, or very hot baths are ineffective, and with the more liberal attitudes to induced abortion which exist today in many countries, only the uninformed try such remedies. Within medicine,

a group of drugs is now available which will induce abortion, but they have to be given with care. These are the ★prostaglandins. In early pregnancy (before the 9th week) prostaglandin pessaries placed high in the vagina usually (but not always) lead to abortion. Later in pregnancy (from the 15th week onwards), prostaglandin injected into the ★amniotic sac, or between the sac and the lining of the uterus, induces an abortion 12 to 36 hours later.

Abortion, induced

The changes which have taken place in people's attitudes, and in the laws in many countries, have meant that induced abortion is now an acceptable way of terminating an unwanted pregnancy. A legally induced abortion is referred to as 'termination of pregnancy'. Most people agree that it is better to prevent an unwanted pregnancy, by remaining chaste or by using appropriate contraceptives, but acknowledge that pregnancy may occur, either because the woman (or her partner) failed to use contraceptives, or because contraception failed. The woman then has to choose between continuing the pregnancy and keeping the baby, or having him adopted, or seeking to have

the pregnancy terminated by an induced abortion. In spite of what is sometimes said, the great majority of women think very seriously about the emotional and the ethical problems involved before they decide to seek an abortion.

Women have always obtained abortions, even in nations which had, and still have, strict laws against abortion. In many cases the abortion was performed inexpertly in unhygienic conditions, and often resulted in pelvic infection, sterility, or even death. Rich women, with better contacts, could obtain a 'safe' abortion, but poor women were at a disadvantage. In countries where abortion is now legal, the number of back-street, dangerous abortions has almost disappeared. The ability to obtain an abortion legally and without fear and loss of self-respect has been welcomed by women everywhere.

Legal abortion which is performed before the 12th week of pregnancy, in an appropriate place, by a trained doctor is safe. It can be carried out under local anaesthesia, when an injection is made into the cervix, or under general anaesthesia. Usually the fetus and placenta are sucked from the uterus using a suction curette which does not damage the lining. A few women bleed rather heavily in the days after the abortion, but treatment is available; a very small number develop a fever which requires antibiotics. The chance of a woman dying from the effects of an abortion is less than 1 in 100000 – less than that following an injection of penicillin.

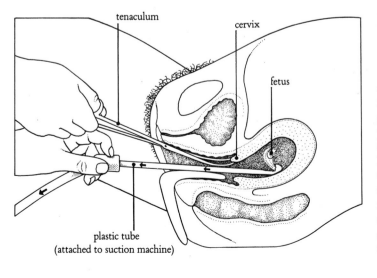

tenaculum

cervix

fetus

plastic tube
(attached to suction machine)

After the 12th week of pregnancy, induced abortion becomes more dangerous. The general practice today is for a quantity of *prostaglandin to be injected into the amniotic sac of fluid which surrounds the fetus. This leads in 12 to 36 hours to an abortion.

Abortion, missed

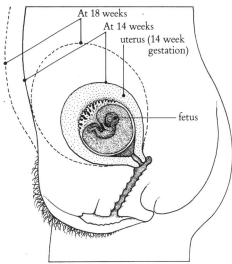

At 18 weeks
At 14 weeks
uterus (14 week gestation)

fetus

In a few cases after a threatened abortion, the bleeding stops and the fetus is not expelled. The symptoms of pregnancy disappear and examination made at intervals reveals that the uterus has ceased to grow. An *ultrasound picture shows that the uterus is filled only with blood clots, or that a small, 'mummified' fetus is present.

There is no urgency in treating a missed abortion, as it is without danger to the woman; she simply needs reassurance that she will not be damaged by having a dead fetus in her body. If an abortion does not occur spontaneously, the doctor, after discussion with the woman and her partner, may decided to induce it. If the uterus is small, he may carry out a *D and C operation to remove the contents, but if it is bigger (larger than the size of a 12-week pregnancy), he may use vaginal pessaries of *prostaglandin or set up an intravenous infusion of dilute prostaglandin. This hormone causes the uterus to contract and expel the dead fetus and placenta.

Abortion, recurrent

A few women among the total number of those who have a spontaneous abortion have recurrent (or habitual) abortions; the figure is put at some 20 per cent. When a woman has had three abortions in succession it is usual for the doctor to establish the shape of the uterus by injecting a radio-opaque substance into it through the cervix, to make sure that it is not congenitally deformed, especially if the abortions have occurred in mid-pregnancy. He will also check that the woman does not have an *incompetent cervix which can cause a late abortion. If neither of these tests shows an abnormality, tests may be carried out on the chromosomes of both partners. If the woman has an abnormally shaped uterus, surgery may help, and treatment is also available for an incompetent cervix. Beyond this there is no validated treatment, although some doctors give hormones, vitamins, and other drugs. One of the problems in evaluating the correct drug treatment is that 3 in 4 women will have a live baby with the next pregnancy.

Abortion, spontaneous

One pregnancy in 15 terminates in spontaneous abortion (or miscarriage), that is the 'products of conception' (the fetus and placenta) are expelled before the 20th week of pregnancy. Abortion may occur spontaneously or may be induced by the action of a doctor or some other person. In some countries, for example Britain, abortion also

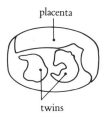

placenta

twins

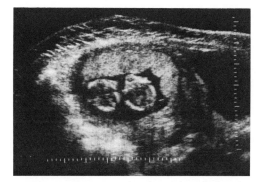

An ultrasound picture may be taken to show the fetus is normal

includes stillborn babies delivered between the 20th and 27th week of pregnancy. Most spontaneous abortions occur in the first 10 weeks, and in about 60 per cent of cases the fetus has failed to develop normally.

The first sign that all is not well is often that slight bleeding occurs. This is called a 'threatened abortion'. Three-quarters of women threatening to abort will go on to have a normal baby. In the remaining cases the pregnancy will be aborted ('inevitable abortion'). There is no specific treatment for threatened abortion and drugs do not help, except perhaps a sedative to reduce anxiety. Most women threatening to abort are asked to stay in bed, but there is no proof that this is of any value. Some doctors measure the level in the blood of a placental protein called human placental lactogen or another called SP1 in an attempt to decide whether the pregnancy will continue or if an abortion will occur.

If the bleeding persists, the doctor may arrange for an *ultrasound picture of the uterus which will show whether the fetus has been formed properly and is living. Most women who are going to abort have bleeding and cramp-like uterine pains, which lead sooner or later to the expulsion of the fetus and placenta. If, as often occurs, the contents of the uterus are not completely expelled ('incomplete abortion'), a *D and C operation may be necessary.

A woman who has aborted spontaneously is usually anxious about the outcome of her next pregnancy. The chance of an abortion recurring is only one in 5. In over 80 per cent of cases the next pregnancy will result in the birth of a live, healthy baby.

Abstinence

Abstinence – abstaining from an action – means, with respect to sex, abstaining from sexual intercourse, although other methods of *sexual pleasuring can be enjoyed. The purpose of sexual abstinence is to enable the woman to remain a virgin, or if she has had sexual intercourse to enable her to avoid becoming pregnant. Permanent abstinence, which includes avoidance of most or all methods of sexual pleasuring, is termed *chastity, and is considered by some religious groups to be expected of those who dedicate their lives to God. Periodic abstinence, which is carried out during those days of the menstrual cycle when the woman is fertile (around the time ovulation occurs), forms the basis of *natural methods of family planning.

Acne

At puberty, there is an increase in the activity of the grease-producing (sebaceous) glands of the skin. The increased activity is probably due to the effects of the sex hormones, particularly *androgens, which are now being produced in the body. As well as producing more grease (sebum) in the gland itself, for some reason the cells lining the duct which connects the gland to the surface of the skin start multiplying, with the result that the duct narrows and may become blocked. If this occurs, a whitehead is formed. On the other hand, if the duct remains open, although narrowed, the gland continues to expand as more sebum is produced, and the duct fills with sebum which dries, forming a

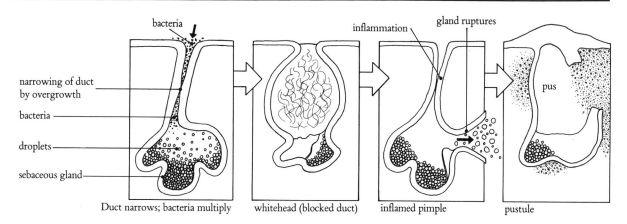

narrowing of duct
by overgrowth

bacteria

droplets

sebaceous gland

bacteria

inflammation

gland ruptures

pus

Duct narrows; bacteria multiply   whitehead (blocked duct)   inflamed pimple   pustule

keratin plug. When the keratin plug meets the air, it turns black. The result is a blackhead which, although unsightly, can be controlled by gentle removal.

Whiteheads are the cause of many of the problems and much of the unsightliness of acne. The gland continues to produce sebum, which cannot escape because the duct is blocked. Inside the gland bacteria called *Propionibacterium acne* act on the sebum, converting some of it to irritating fatty acids. Eventually the gland bursts, expelling the fatty acids (and bacteria) into the surrounding tissue. This results in a pustule or, if deeper in the skin, in a tender, inflamed pimple. Some of these pustules and swellings are converted into scar-tissue during the healing process, leaving the pits sometimes seen on the face or neck of an acne sufferer.

Acne occurs most commonly on the face, chest, shoulders, and back, and it can be aggravated by emotional stress. Its presence can, in turn, cause great emotional distress, particularly as the condition is more common during adolescence, when between 60 and 80 per cent of teenagers are affected, 15 per cent severely. Acne usually ceases by the age of 25, but some continue to develop new lesions of acne into their thirties or forties.

Acne is not caused by eating rich or fatty foods, and dietary restrictions, such as cutting out sugar or fats, have proved ineffective. Acne is not due to poor personal hygiene, to lack of exercise, to overindulgence in alcohol, or to masturbation.

Until recently, the treatment for acne has been relatively unsatisfactory and even today

there is no single prescribed regimen. The principles of treatment are firstly, to reduce the numbers of bacteria (and fatty acids) in the glands; secondly, to contain the excessive growth of the cells lining the ducts; and finally, to eliminate the whiteheads, pustules, and nodules.

Acne can be controlled, to some extent, if the person regularly uses soap to wash the affected area and, if possible, scrubs the skin gently using a soft brush. If acne affects the face, thick make-up should be avoided and a non-medicated, lightweight, non-greasy make-up chosen. If the acne is bad the psychological benefit of using make-up may be considerable.

Mild acne generally only needs to be treated with medications applied to the affected areas of the skin. Two drugs are available for these purposes, benzyl peroxide and retinoic acid. Both are potentially irritating and must only be used under strict medical supervision. Benzyl peroxide inhibits the growth of *P.acne* and reduces the production of fatty acids in the gland; retinoic acid makes the cells of the ducts less adhesive, so that they are shed from the lining and the blocked ducts reopen. The drugs are available in the form of a jelly, cream, or lotion, which is applied to the affected area of skin. The treatment has to be continued for 3 to 6 months to clear up the acne, and continuing supervision is needed in severe cases.

If the person has a great many pustules, antibiotics are often prescribed. The usual ones are tetracycline or erythromycin; these are both relatively cheap and free from side-effects. As it takes up to 3 weeks for the antibiotic to penetrate the glands, tetracycline has to be given for a minimum of 4 weeks and often for 2 to 4 months. Tetracycline should be taken one hour before eating, not with food, as food prevents it from being absorbed.

Another form of treatment which is recommended is to prescribe oestrogens, which reduce the production rate of sebum. Oestrogens are usually given in the form of the contraceptive *pill, and the doctor chooses a combination containing rather more oestrogen than is normally given for contraceptive purposes. With this treatment it usually takes 2 or 3 months before the acne clears. In more severe cases the doctor may prescribe oestrogen together with an anti-androgen drug, called cyproterone.

How should a girl who has acne be treated? The first treatment should be either benzyl peroxide or antibiotics. If no improvement occurs over a period of 3 months, an oral contraceptive pill should be tried. If no improvement occurs over a 6-month period, then at this stage retinoic acid or the oestrogen–cyproterone combination should be prescribed.

Adolescence

Adolescence is defined in *The Oxford English Dictionary* as the period between childhood and maturity extending from 14 to 25 in males and 12 to 21 in females. It is a period of both physical and psychological growth. During adolescence a girl's body undergoes a number of profound changes and develops from that of a child to that of a woman; this period of physical growth is known as *puberty. The onset of menstruation occurs (*menarche), and the menstrual periods gradually become regular and rhythmic. These physical changes are due to the female sex hormone, oestrogen, which is circulating in the blood. There is considerable variation among girls in the age at which the increase in height, the development of the breasts, the appearance of pubic hair, and the onset of menstruation occur, but in general terms girls mature a year or two earlier than boys. It has been observed that late maturers (both girls and boys) are less attractive physically to others, less well poised, less popular with their peers, and more likely to seek attention than early maturers.

The psychological changes of adolescence are many and varied. It is a time when learning capacity is at its peak and when reasoning becomes clearer; the adolescent begins to make decisions, to choose with discrimination, and to become aware of what is possible and what is fantasy. During this period, which is often characterized by confusion and uncertainty, the adolescent seeks to find her identity, to answer the question 'Who am I?' In this search, she may reject parental values, but none the less needs some parental direction and the opportunity to talk with her parents. The influence of her peers will inevitably affect her behaviour, and gentle discipline from her parents may be necessary so that the adjustment to adulthood may take place smoothly.

The circulating sex hormones also initiate sexual fantasies, and sexual arousal is common. This results in vaginal lubrication, which may cause the girl anxiety, if she finds her pants are stained. Many teenage girls masturbate, which is healthy and, as well as being pleasurable, gives the girl the opportunity to explore her body.

Today many teenagers are sexually active. Surveys carried out in Britain, Scandinavia, and the United States have shown that the proportion of sexually active teenage girls increases from 25 per cent at the age of 16 to 70 per cent at the age of 19. Only a few girls are promiscuous, and the great majority have a relationship with a single partner which usually lasts for a period of months, or even longer. However, increased sexual activity is associated with an increase both in teenage pregnancy and in *sexually transmitted diseases. If an unmarried teenager becomes pregnant, the consequences are serious. Either she will seek an *abortion, or she will have the baby as a single girl (and will either keep the baby or have it adopted), or she will marry and have the baby. Each decision is difficult. Pregnancy can usually be avoided if sexually active teenagers take advantage of family planning services. Pregnancy in a teenager poses few obstetrical problems, provided the girl receives adequate antenatal care, but the psychological problems of bearing and rearing a child may be considerable.

Adoption

Couples who, after investigation, are unable to have a child may find both the solution to their problem and personal fulfilment by adopting one or more children. Other couples who already have children of their own may choose to look after, and eventually adopt, a handicapped or deprived child. Following the legal process of adoption, the adoptive couple become the child's father and mother and have both the responsibilities and rewards of that status. In many Western countries the number of children available for adoption is becoming increasingly limited, as more single pregnant women (or married women with several children) choose either to have an abortion or to give birth and keep the child.

Before any couple are accepted as clients for adoption, both partners have to agree to be scrutinized medically and psychologically to confirm that they are fit to adopt a child. Once accepted, they are placed on a waiting list until a child has been surrended by its mother to the adoption agency and is available for adoption.

As the number of children available for adoption has fallen, couples may have to wait for up to five years to adopt. Adoption of a small baby causes few problems, but the adoption of a child who has been in an institution for some time may not be easy, as the child has to adjust to a new environment. A couple who choose to adopt a child not only give that child the warmth of their relationship, but receive from the child pleasure and pride. Of course, as in families who have naturally born children, problems may arise, but there is no evidence that these are more frequent or more severe when the child has been adopted. After adopting the child, the parents have the responsibility of telling the child at an appropriate time that he or she has been adopted. In some countries the child has the right to know and meet his or her natural mother.

In most Western countries adoption can only be made through a recognized adoption agency, and prospective parents should beware of dealing with any other organization or individual.

Adrenogenital syndrome

A small number of babies (mostly female) are born with external genitals which are ambiguous, resembling in part those of both sexes. The most common cause of ambiguous genitals in a female is a congenital defect of a group of enzymes which prevent the production of the hormone cortisone. This condition induces the adrenal gland to produce the male hormone androgen, with the result that the baby is born with an enlarged clitoris, which looks like a small penis. The adrenogenital syndrome tends to run in families, with other female children being affected. If a child is born with ambiguous genitals, a swab is taken from the inside of its

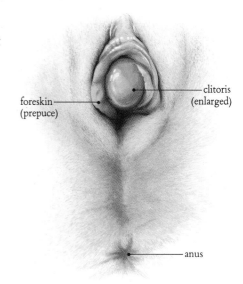

foreskin
(prepuce)

clitoris
(enlarged)

anus

cheek to see if the cells have ★Barr bodies, which indicate the baby is female. The levels of hormones and electrolytes in the baby's blood are measured, and cortisone is given to correct the defect. The abnormally large clitoris is treated surgically when the child is 3 or 4 years old. Often surgical treatment to open the vagina is necessary as a teenager.

After-pains

In the first days after childbirth, a mother may complain of cramp-like uterine pain, which may become strong, particularly when she suckles her baby. The pains are due to contractions of the muscle of the uterus, in response to the release of the hormone ★oxytocin from the pituitary gland. The treatment is to prescribe aspirin or one of the anti-prostaglandin drugs. In severe cases an injection of pethidine may be needed. The after-pains will normally cease within a few days of giving birth.

Ageing

To grow old is inevitable, but to feel old is not, and is very much a state of mind. Physical ageing occurs in all body systems. The senses become less acute, hearing decreases and higher-pitched notes can be heard less easily, so that some degree of deafness affects about 25 per cent of people aged 70. The sharpness of sight decreases and the ability to focus easily diminishes. The sense of smell also declines or changes. Teeth tend to be less firmly fixed. The hair becomes grey and then white. After the age of 70, the body's temperature control becomes less efficient, and cold is felt more intensely. Manual dexterity diminishes, clumsiness increases, and the muscles begin to lose their power. Illnesses, such as ★high blood pressure, ★rheumatism, stroke, heart disease, and cancer become more frequent, as does ★osteoporosis.

In spite of increasing disabilities, however, people do not need to *feel* old. People tend to feel old, either because they have abused their bodies over the years by excessive food, or alcohol, or cigarettes, or too little exercise, or because they believe the myth that old people are inferior, no longer have any real value, and should behave according to an expected pattern. A wise man said, 'I will never be an old man. To me, old age is always fifteen years older than I am.' And a wise woman wrote, 'In old age we should wish to have passions strong enough to prevent us turning in on ourselves. One's life has values so long as one attributes value to the life of others, by means of love, friendship, indignation, compassion.'

The physical and mental effects of ageing can be reduced if older people take the following simple measures:

Have periodic checks by a doctor who is interested in ageing

Eat a prudent ★diet

Exercise moderately and regularly

Remain curious about life and passionate about causes

Continue to keep the mind exercised

In Western societies, women tend to live longer than men so that a disproportionate number of elderly people are female. Many of these elderly women are lonely, often poor, and occasionally malnourished. Society is increasingly aware of the problems of the elderly, but action to change the existing situation is only likely to occur if older people become more vocal and assertive on their own behalf.

Ageing and sexuality

When a woman reaches the menopause she can no longer reproduce, but she can continue to enjoy her sexuality into old age. She continues to have sexual desires, to be sexually aroused, and also to respond to sexual stimulus. The myth that older women are sexually neutral is without foundation, as many women have greater sexual desire, and obtain greater sexual pleasure, after the menopause than before.

With the advent of the *menopause, the ovaries cease to produce female sex hormones, and there is a considerable drop in the level of oestrogen circulating in the blood, although a varying amount of oestrogen is produced in other parts of the body. The withdrawal of oestrogen leads to a decrease in size of the genital organs. The lining of the vagina may become thinner, making intercourse painful, although regular sexual intercourse will prevent this. If intercourse does become painful, then the use of oestrogen cream, inserted into the vagina in accordance with a doctor's directions, will be found to be helpful.

After the menopause, a woman's sexual response alters. Her nipples respond less readily to sexual stimulation, and there is a lesser degree of clitoral enlargement and genital swelling. Vaginal lubrication is also slower and the quantity is diminished. A woman may take longer to reach orgasm and it may be less intense. However, this varies from woman to woman.

The frequency with which an older woman both desires and enjoys sex depends on her attitude to sexuality when she was younger. The more she enjoyed sex in her youth, the more likely she is to enjoy it as she grows older. The crucial factor is her relationship with her partner. If the couple enjoy cuddling, touching, and other forms of physical contact, the woman will obtain sexual pleasure and this will be enhanced if the couple choose to have sexual intercourse. Studies in the United States have shown that over 70 per cent of couples have regular sexual intercourse in their late sixties, and that 10 per cent still enjoy intercourse in their eighties. When sexual intercourse ceases it is usually because the man is no longer able or willing because of infirmity, illness, or age. However, the woman can be sexually stimulated in other ways by her partner.

As women live longer than men, there are proportionally more widowed women than widowed men. Some widows may form new relationships, others live contentedly having adjusted to their new status, and still others become unhappy as they continue to have sexual needs but have no partner with whom to form a relationship. Some women solve the problem by masturbating, others would like to masturbate but feel that they require 'permission' to do so from a doctor. Sympathetic counselling and advice will help those women dispel any feelings they may have of guilt or doubt.

Alcohol in pregnancy

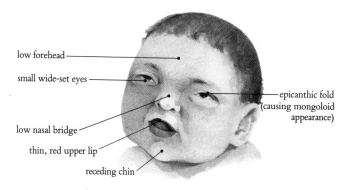

low forehead

small wide-set eyes

epicanthic fold (causing mongoloid appearance)

low nasal bridge

thin, red upper lip

receding chin

The consumption of alcohol in pregnancy may lead to a baby affected by the fetal alcohol syndrome. At birth the baby is underweight, has delayed development, and may have some degree of mental retardation. Abuse of alcohol in pregnancy may also increase the chance of an abortion occurring. For these reasons, it is advisable for a pregnant woman to avoid alcohol altogether or, if that is impossible, to restrict herself to a glass of wine or beer taken occasionally with a meal.

Amenorrhoea

Amenorrhoea is the name given to the condition when a woman fails to have menstrual periods. The condition is known as 'primary amenorrhoea' when the woman has never menstruated; and as 'secondary amenorrhoea' if her periods cease after having been regular for some months or years. The most common cause of amenorrhoea is pregnancy and this is always excluded before other possible causes are considered.

Secondary amenorrhoea is not usually investigated until the periods have been absent for about 9 to 12 months, as in many instances they return spontaneously during this time. Medical research has refined the type of investigations which are required. The woman's weight is noted, as women who have lost weight because of severe dieting or because of *anorexia nervosa often have amenorrhoea, and this responds not to medication but to a gain in weight. An X-ray is made of the skull to exclude any tumour of the pituitary area. If the X-ray suggests a tumour, a CAT (computerized axial tomograph) scan is performed. The machine uses a computer to build up clear cross-sections of the pituitary at different levels. The technique enables the doctor to see the area of the pituitary with greater clarity than an ordinary X-ray. Blood tests are taken to measure the pituitary hormone *FSH, *prolactin, and thyroid-stimulating hormone. The woman is given a hormone tablet (*gestagen) to be taken twice daily for 5 days. If this course of medication is followed by a menstrual period, it indicates that her ovaries are functioning.

With the information obtained from these tests, which can be made during one or two visits, the doctor can determine the cause of the amenorrhoea and can recommend treatment if the woman wants it. Treatment is usually only requested if the woman wishes to become pregnant. Amenorrhoea in itself causes no harm to the woman and may spare her the inconvenience of menstruating.

Amniocentesis

Amniocentesis is the withdrawal of a sample of fluid from the *amniotic sac which surrounds the fetus. The position of the fetus is determined by *ultrasound and then with local anaesthetic a long needle is pushed through the abdominal wall into the amniotic sac, avoiding the fetus and the placenta.

Amniocentesis is performed at about the 15th week of pregnancy in women who have given birth to babies with *neural tube defects, or whose previous babies have had certain inherited *metabolic diseases. It is also carried out at this time in pregnant women over the age of 35 to find out if the fetus has *Down's syndrome (mongolism).

In mid-pregnancy, amniocentesis is carried out on women who have *Rhesus isoimmune disease and whose blood has been found to contain antibodies. The sample is examined on a machine which indicates the severity of the condition and whether the fetus needs a transfusion in the uterus. In late pregnancy a sample of fluid may be taken before labour is induced, to determine whether the baby's lungs are sufficiently mature to avoid the development of *hyaline membrane disease.

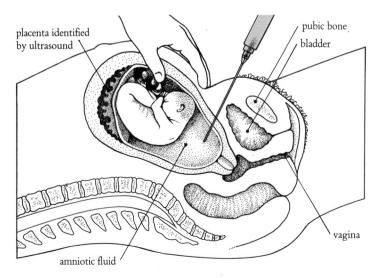

placenta identified by ultrasound

pubic bone

bladder

vagina

amniotic fluid

Amniotic sac and fluid
Anaemia, iron-deficiency
Anaemias, vitamin-deficiency

Amniotic sac and fluid

The fetus lives almost weightless in a bag of water – the amniotic sac – which fills the cavity of the uterus. Like an astronaut it floats, moves, kicks, 'breathes', sucks its fingers, and hears and responds to noise. It is protected by the amniotic fluid from injury and is maintained at a constant temperature. Its only connection to its 'life-support system' – the *placenta – is the *umbilical cord. Fluid appears in the primitive sac as early as five days after conception, and increases rapidly from the 10th week of pregnancy. By the 30th week, the sac contains the fetus (which now weighs 1200 g) and 600 ml of amniotic fluid (*liquor amnii*). The maximum amount of 1000 ml is reached at 35 weeks, after which the fluid declines to 600 ml at 40 weeks.

The amniotic fluid is not like a stagnant pond: it is constantly changing. The fetus swallows some of the fluid which then enters the fetal circulation. As the fetal kidneys become active, the fetus urinates into the amniotic sac, and in late pregnancy fluid is added from the fetal circulation through its skin. The cells covering the placenta also add to the volume of the amniotic sac.

The amniotic sac and fluid are the 'bag of waters' which is ruptured to herald the onset of labour (see *Childbirth, labour).

Anaemia, iron-deficiency

Iron-deficiency anaemia is the most common of the various kinds of anaemia that are encountered in women in developed countries. Iron is required to make haem, the pigment present in the red blood cells which carries oxygen to the tissues. Every day millions of red blood cells die, releasing iron which is taken up by the new red blood cells formed in the bone marrow. Iron is also lost in sweat, in the cells shed constantly by the skin, and in menstrual blood. Unless the iron is replaced by iron obtained from food, anaemia will result after a period of time. Most healthy women eat a prudent *diet which provides sufficient iron, but a few, who indulge in *binge-eating or eat junk foods, may become iron-deficient, and develop anaemia. A few women who have heavy menstrual bleeding may become anaemic if the condition persists for several months. Anaemia may also occur in pregnancy because the fetus requires iron; but if the diet is nutritious and well balanced this is unlikely.

Anaemia is more common among elderly women, whose diet tends to be poor, and among women who abuse analgesic tablets (particularly aspirin), as these cause minor haemorrhages in the stomach. Mild anaemia is generally only discovered by testing the blood, as it does not cause pallor, tiredness, or breathlessness. The treatment is simple. The woman takes iron tablets by mouth, and only in special circumstances are iron injections or blood transfusion needed. Anaemia can usually be avoided if a nutritious, well-balanced diet is eaten.

Anaemias, vitamin-deficiency

Vitamin-deficiency (megaloblastic) anaemias, which may be found in association with *iron-deficiency anaemia, are most often caused by a lack of vitamin B_{12} or a lack of folate. The blood cells become larger than normal, so that when a sample of blood is examined under a microscope megaloblasts are seen (megalo = big; blasts = a type of blood cell).

Vitamin B_{12} anaemia, which is known as *pernicious anaemia*, is more common among older women. It is caused by a deficiency of the protein secreted in the stomach which is needed for the absorption of vitamin B_{12}, or because of certain bowel diseases. Very old people whose diet lacks the vitamin may also develop pernicious anaemia. The treatment is to give monthly injections of vitamin B_{12}.

Anaemias, vitamin-deficiency
Anal intercourse
Anatomy, female genital

Folate-deficiency anaemia is found in pregnant women and among poor people, mainly in the developing countries. It is due to a lack of folic acid in the diet. A good source of folic acid is green leafy vegetables. The drug phenytoin (Dilantin or Epineutin), used to control epilepsy, is another cause of this type of anaemia.

Anal intercourse

One of the ways in which male homosexuals obtain sexual pleasure is anal sex, when one partner inserts his penis into the anus and rectum of the other. The legal term for anal intercourse is buggery or sodomy, and it remains a felony in most Western countries, even between consenting parties. Anal intercourse also occurs in heterosexual relationships, but the number of couples who use this sexual variation is unknown, and is probably less than 10 per cent. In some subcultures anal intercourse is practised as a method of birth control, when religious beliefs or poverty bar the use of contraceptives.

The anal area is a highly erotic region of the body and many people enjoy it being stimulated by hand or mouth during *sexual pleasuring; however, this does not normally lead to anal intercourse. In a loving sexual relationship, anal intercourse may be enjoyed by both partners, but often it appears that the man insists on anal intercourse without his partner's consent, either because he is drunk or is hostile and wishes to degrade the woman, or because he believes he will obtain more sexual pleasure by forcing his penis through the relatively tight muscle ring surrounding the anus. When anal intercourse takes place in a loving relationship it means that both partners consent to and enjoy this form of sexual pleasuring. Unlike the vagina which lubricates when a woman is aroused sexually, the anus remains dry, and for comfort the man must put a lubricant (saliva, jelly, cream, or butter) around and inside his partner's anus and on his penis.

Unless anal intercourse takes place frequently, penetration must be slow, as the anal muscle goes into spasm when touched and takes some 20 seconds or longer to relax. Many women find penetration uncomfortable, but once the penis is inside the anus enjoy the experience of thrusting, which must be gentle. With experience, the duration of the spasm and the amount of discomfort are reduced. A penis thrusting inside the anal canal will not do any damage, and once it is withdrawn the anal muscle contracts – stories of anal damage are untrue.

Apart from the legal prohibition on anal intercourse, it is associated with some medical problems. The lower bowel is heavily contaminated with bacteria which may infect the man's urethra, or if he follows anal intercourse with vaginal penetration, the woman's vagina may be infected. To avoid any risk of infection, the man should pass urine after anal intercourse and wash his penis with soap and water before engaging in other forms of sexual pleasuring.

Anatomy, female genital

Unlike the genital organs of the male, most of the female genital organs lie inside the body, hidden from view. Because of this many woman have never looked at their external genitals, using a mirror, and have never touched them, and are therefore ignorant about this important part of their own anatomy.

The external genital organs The anatomical name for the external genitals is the *vulva*. It is made up of several structures which surround the entrance to the vagina, each of which has its own separate function. The *labia majora* (the large lips of the vagina) are two large folds of skin which contain sweat glands and hair follicles embedded in fat. The size of the labia majora varies considerably. In infancy and in old age they are small, and the fat is not present; in the reproductive years, between puberty and the menopause, they are well filled with fatty tissue. In front (looked at from between the legs), they join together in the pad of fat which surmounts the pelvic bone, and which is called the 'mount of Venus' (*mons veneris*). Both of the labia, and more particularly the *mons veneris*, are covered with hair, the quantity of which varies from woman to woman. The pubic hair on the abdominal side of the *mons veneris* usually terminates in a straight line, but may simulate the male hair-line which stretches upwards in an inverted 'V' to reach the umbilicus. The inner surfaces of the labia majora are free from hair, and are separated by a small groove from the thin labia minora, which guard the entrance to the vagina.

The *labia minora* (the small lips of the vagina) are delicate folds of skin which contain little fatty tissue. They vary in size, and in front split into two folds, one of which passes over and the other under the clitoris. At the back they join to form the fourchette, which often tears during childbirth. In the reproductive years, the labia minora are partly hidden by the labia majora, but in childhood and old age the labia minora appear more prominent because the labia majora are relatively small. The fold of the labia minora which passes over the clitoris is equivalent to the male foreskin (prepuce). The fold of skin (the frenulum) which passes under the clitoris is the equivalent of the small band of tissue which joins the pink glans of the penis to the skin which covers it.

The *clitoris* lies in a fold of the inner lips of the vulva, in front of the pubic bone. Its size varies considerably, but is usually that of a green pea. It is about 2 cm in length, and becomes erect on sexual stimulation. Most of the clitoris can only be felt if it is pressed against the pubic bone, but its tip (or glans) is visible under the labial fold which is also called the clitoral hood. The clitoris has the same origin in the embryo as the penis and, in many ways, is its female equivalent. It is made up of erectile tissue which fills with blood on stimulation and has a rich supply of nerves. Stimulation of the clitoris either indirectly during sexual intercourse or directly by gentle stroking of the clitoral area by finger or tongue increases a woman's sexual arousal. Many women who are unable to

reach orgasm during sexual intercourse do so easily and enjoyably by self-stimulation of the clitoris or if their partner stimulates the clitoris using a finger or the tongue. In sexual intercourse, the movement of the man's penis in the vagina indirectly stimulates the clitoris and can lead to the woman having an orgasm. As sexual excitement mounts, the clitoris increases in size.

The cleft below the clitoris and between the labia minora is called the *vestibule* (or entrance). Just below the clitoris is the external opening of the urethra, the part of the urinary tract which connects the bladder to the outside. In old women the urethral orifice may stretch, and the lining of the lower part of the urethra may be exposed.

Below the external urethral orifice is the *hymen*, which surrounds the vaginal orifice. The hymen is a thin, incomplete fold of membrane with one or more apertures. It varies considerably in shape and in elasticity, but is generally stretched or torn during the first attempt at sexual intercourse. The tearing is usually followed by a minute amount of bleeding. In many cultures the rupture of the hymen (also called the maidenhead), and the consequent bleeding, was considered a sign that the girl was a virgin at the time of marriage, and the bed was inspected on the morning after the first night of the honeymoon for evidence of blood. Although an 'intact' hymen is considered a sign of virginity, it is not a reliable sign, as in some cases sexual intercourse fails to cause a tear, and in others the hymen may have been torn previously by exploring fingers, either of the girl herself or of her sexual partner. The stretching and tearing of the hymen at the first intercourse may be painful, particularly if the partners are apprehensive or ignorant of sexual matters; if the couple is relaxed with each other, the discomfort is minimal. Childbirth causes a much greater tearing of the hymen, and after delivery only a few tags remain, called *carunculae myrtiformes*. Just outside the hymen, still within the vestibule but deep beneath the skin, are two collections of erectile tissues which fill with blood during sexual arousal. Deep in the backward part of the vestibule are two pea-sized glands which also secrete mucus during sexual

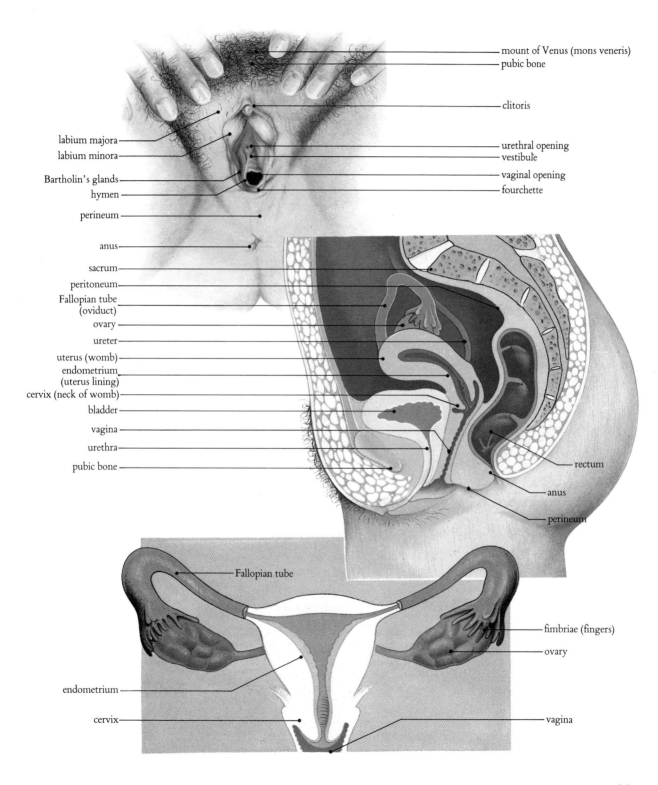

mount of Venus (mons veneris)
pubic bone

clitoris

labium majora
labium minora

urethral opening
vestibule

Bartholin's glands
hymen

vaginal opening
fourchette

perineum

anus

sacrum

peritoneum

Fallopian tube
(oviduct)

ovary

ureter

uterus (womb)

endometrium
(uterus lining)

cervix (neck of womb)

bladder

vagina

urethra

pubic bone

rectum

anus

perineum

Fallopian tube

fimbriae (fingers)

ovary

endometrium

cervix

vagina

arousal and moisten the entrance to the vagina, so that the penis may enter it without discomfort. They are known as *Bartholin's glands*, and can become infected.

The area of the vulva between the posterior fourchette and the anus, and the muscles under the skin, form a pyramid-shaped wedge of tissue separating the vagina and the rectum. It is called the *perineum, and is of considerable importance in childbirth as the muscles have to stretch to enable the fetus to be born. In many cases, the tissues tear or an incision called an *episiotomy is made to avoid this occurring.

The internal genital organs The internal genital organs consist of the vagina, the uterus, the Fallopian tubes (or oviducts), and the ovaries. The *vagina* is a muscular tube which stretches upwards and backwards from the vestibule to reach the uterus. As well as being muscular, it contains a well-developed network of veins which become distended in sexual arousal. Normally, the walls of the vagina lie close together. The vagina is a potential cavity which is distended by intravaginal tampons used during menstruation, by the penis at intercourse, and during childbirth, when it can stretch very considerably to permit the baby to be born. The vagina is about 9 cm long, and at the upper end the cervix (or neck) of the uterus projects into it. The vagina lies between the bladder in front and the rectum (or back-passage) behind. At the sides it is surrounded and protected by the strong muscles of the floor of the pelvis. Unless the vagina has been damaged, injured, or tightened as a result of surgery, or has not developed due to an absence of sex hormones, its size is quite adequate for sexual intercourse. The woman who menstruates has a normal-sized vagina, and 'difficulty' at intercourse may simply be due to inadequate sexual arousal.

The vagina is a remarkable organ. Not only is it capable of great distension, but it keeps itself clean. The walls of the vagina are formed by cells which lie on each other in layers 30 cells deep like the bricks of a house wall. In the reproductive years, the top layer of cells is constantly being shed into the vagina, where they are acted upon by a small bacillus which normally lives there, to produce lactic acid. The lactic acid kills any contaminating germs which may happen to get into the vagina. Because of this self-cleansing process, it is unnecessary to use vaginal douches. In childhood, the wall of the vagina is thin, and the production of lactic acid does not take place. However, this is of little importance, because the vagina is not usually contaminated at this age. In old age, the lining becomes thin again, and few cells are shed. This means that little or no lactic acid is formed, and contaminating germs may grow, which sometimes results in inflammation of the vagina.

The *uterus* (or womb) is a hollow, muscular organ which averages 9 cm in length, 6 cm in width at its widest point, and weighs 60 g. In pregnancy, it enlarges to weigh 1000 g, and is able to contain a baby measuring 40 cm in length. It is able to undergo these changes because of the complex structure of its muscle and its exceptional response to the female sex hormones. The uterus is located in the middle of the bony pelvis, lying between the bladder in front and the bowel behind. It is pear-shaped, and its muscular front and back walls bulge into the cavity which is normally narrow and slit-like, until pregnancy occurs. Viewed from the front, the cavity is triangular, and is lined with a special tissue made up of glands in a network of cells. This tissue is called the *endometrium*, and it undergoes changes during each menstrual cycle. For descriptive purposes, the uterus is divided into an upper part (or body) and a lower part (or cervix uteri: the neck of the uterus). The *cervix* projects into the upper part of the vagina. The cavity of the uterus is narrow in the cervix, where it is called the cervical canal; it is widest in the body of the uterus, and then narrows again towards the cornu (or horn), where the cavity is continuous with the hollow of the Fallopian tube.

The lower part of the uterus and the upper part of the cervix are supported by a sling of special tissues, called the cardinal ligament, which are attached to the muscles of the pelvic wall like a fan. These supports may be stretched in childbirth, leading to a *prolapse later in life. With improved obstetrics and better education for childbirth this complication is much less common today.

Normally the uterus lies bent forwards at an angle of 90° to the vagina, resting on the bladder. As the bladder fills, it rotates backwards; as it empties, the uterus falls forward. In about 10 per cent of women the uterus lies bent backwards. This is called retroversion. (See also ★Retroverted uterus.)

The *Fallopian tubes* (or oviducts) are two small, hollow tubes which stretch for about 10 cm from the upper part of the uterus, one on each side, to lie in contact with the ovary. The outer end of each Fallopian tube is divided into long finger-like processes called fimbriae, and it is thought that these sweep up the egg when it is expelled from the ovary. The tube is lined with cells shaped like goblets, which lie between cells with frond-like borders. The Fallopian tube is of great importance, as this is where fertilization of the egg takes place, and it is likely that its secretions help to nourish the fertilized egg as

it is transported by the wafting movements of the fronds towards the uterus.

The *ovaries* (or gonads) are two ovoid-shaped organs averaging 3.5 cm in length and 2 cm in width. In the infant they are small, delicate, thin structures, but after puberty they enlarge to reach full size. After the ★menopause they become small and wrinkled, and in old age are less than half their adult size. Each ovary has a centre made up of small cells and a mesh of vessels. Surrounding this is the ovary proper (the cortex) containing about 200 000 egg cells (ova) which lie in a cellular bed (the stroma). The egg cells and the stroma are protected by a thickened layer of tissue. The ovaries are the equivalent of the male testes, and in addition to containing the egg cells on which all human life depends they are also a hormone factory which produces the vital female sex hormones.

Androgens

An androgen is one of the group of male sex hormones, of which testosterone is the most important. Androgens are produced mainly in a man's testicles, though a small quantity is produced in the adrenal glands. At puberty the concentration of testosterone in the blood increases, and this leads to growth of the penis and testicles, and to the development of the male physique. Hair grows on the man's face and body, his voice deepens, his Adam's apple becomes more prominent, his shoulders become broader, and his muscles increase in size. Androgens are also involved in triggering a man's sexual drive (sexual desire and arousal). As a man grows older the quantity of testosterone decreases, but it

remains at a level sufficient to maintain his sexuality until old age.

Women also produce small quantities of androgens in their adrenal glands, but any effect (apart from triggering sexual drive) is masked by the effects of the female sex hormone, ★oestrogen, which is produced in large amounts. A few women develop a tumour of the adrenal gland or a particular ovarian tumour, either of which may secrete androgens. If this occurs, the woman's clitoris grows larger, hair may appear on her face, her voice may deepen, and her breasts may become smaller. These changes are called ★virilization. If the tumour is removed surgically, the signs of virilization regress.

Anorexia nervosa

Anorexia nervosa is an illness which occurs most frequently in women. It usually starts in adolescence or the early twenties, and affects one woman in every 100 under the age of 25 in the developed nations. A woman who has anorexia nervosa fears that she will become fat and that she will lose control over

her eating. She starts on a relentless pursuit of thinness.

Most women with anorexia nervosa begin losing weight by dieting strictly, sometimes combining this with excessive exercise. A number of women later resort to more dangerous methods of losing weight such as self-induced vomiting or the excessive use of laxatives or diuretics.

The victim of anorexia nervosa aims to lose weight. Her weight usually falls to at least 80 per cent of the average for her age and height, and in most cases the fall is much greater and the emaciation extreme. In addition, menstruation ceases, and she may develop one or more of a number of physical problems. These include a slow heart rate, low blood pressure, tiredness, cold hands and feet, and perhaps the appearance of soft downy hair on her arms, face, and back. There may be disturbances of her body electrolytes, which can be dangerous to life.

Often the woman wishes to increase her body weight by a small amount, but fears that if she eats more, or gives up her weight-losing behaviours, she will lose control and become fat. In some anorexia nervosa patients who also binge-eat (★bulimia), this fear may become a reality.

The illness requires treatment, but many sufferers deny that they are ill, and may refuse to be treated until they feel that they really need it. A few women become very ill and require urgent admission to hospital. The treatment of anorexia nervosa is to restore the woman's body weight to normal, and this is achieved by feeding, under firm control, often in hospital; counselling and psychotherapy are also needed. It may take between 6 months and 6 years before a sufferer is 'cured' and, during this time, periods of normal weight are achieved, with frequent relapses. One anorexic in 5 becomes, or is, a binge-eater, and one in 10 continues to be thin and have an eating disorder throughout her life.

Anorexia nervosa, the 'slimming disease' may follow a period of strict dieting; the woman has an obsessional fear of becoming fat

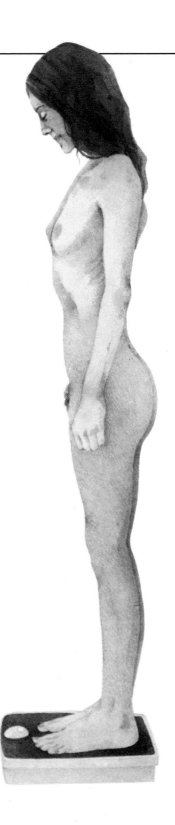

Antenatal care

Antenatal (or prenatal) care, the periodic assessment of the woman and her unborn baby during pregnancy, has several objectives. These are, to ensure that the mother is physically and psychologically as healthy, or healthier, during pregnancy as she was before becoming pregnant; to detect factors occurring during pregnancy which may adversely affect the healthy growth and development of the baby; to educate the mother about the processes of pregnancy and childbirth; and to provide information about nutrition, breast-feeding, adjustment to parenthood, sexuality, and other matters which may affect both the parents and their baby. In essence, antenatal care is preventive medicine: and its acceptance by women, and their partners, has been an important factor in the fall in both the maternal and *perinatal mortality rates which have occurred in most countries in the past fifty years.

The woman's first visit to a doctor *should take place in the first 10 weeks of pregnancy*, so that she may be examined and laboratory tests initiated. The physical examination includes a vaginal examination and the measurement of blood pressure. Laboratory tests are made on samples of urine and blood, and include determination of the blood group (including the rhesus group) and tests to exclude anaemia, diabetes, syphilis, and urinary tract infection.

Pregnant women are usually asked to attend a doctor or a clinic at intervals of 4 to 6 weeks up to the 28th week; at 2-weekly intervals to the 36th week, and then each subsequent week until the baby is born. At each visit the health professional (doctor or nurse) discusses any problems the woman may have, gives advice about general health matters, and examines the woman's abdomen to palpate (feel) the fetus; her blood pressure is also checked and a sample of urine taken. At the 28th and 36th weeks a further blood sample is taken to check that she is not suffering from anaemia.

In the past ten years, *ultrasound techniques have been used increasingly to 'visualize' the fetus. In many centres today a routine ultrasound examination of the pelvis is made at about the 12th week to confirm the duration of the pregnancy; or between the 16th to 20th week for the same purpose, and to determine if the woman is bearing twins. The benefit in terms of cost of routine ultrasound examinations has not been established, but selective examinations have proved valuable.

In some centres all pregnant women are screened by means of a blood test at about the 15th week to determine if the fetus has a *neural tube defect, especially spina bifida. If the test suggests a defect, it is usually repeated, and then further tests are made, including ultrasound assessment and perhaps taking a sample of the amniotic fluid in which the fetus lives (*amniocentesis). An amniocentesis is also carried out on women over the age of 35, who request the test, to detect if the fetus has *Down's syndrome. In the last 4 weeks of pregnancy a further vaginal examination is made to assess the size of both the pelvis and the fetus.

To be fully effective, antenatal care requires the cooperation of the woman and the health professionals. There must be good communication between them based on trust and understanding. The health professional should explain the purpose of any tests which are ordered, and be prepared and willing to answer any questions the woman (or her partner) may have about pregnancy, childbirth, or infant care.

Apareunia

In this condition, the woman is unable to permit the man's penis to enter her vagina, although she may respond to and enjoy other forms of *sexual pleasuring. It happens that in a few instances, the woman may have a local condition, such as *genital herpes, or narrowing of the vagina as a result of disease, but in most cases the cause is psychological. Because of a lack of sexual knowledge or because of rigidly stern attitudes towards sexuality learned during childhood, the woman fears penetration by the man's penis. She may believe that she will be damaged by the penis, or that she is 'small made'. She may dislike the thought of physical sex, and may regard it as indecent.

Treatment involves teaching the woman about her genital anatomy and, with the help of a therapist, convincing her that sexual intercourse is neither dangerous nor indecent. In nearly every case of apareunia treatment is successful.

Apgar score

The most important adjustment a newborn baby has to make is to breathe. Once it is breathing, oxygen is taken into its lungs and the other body systems respond in turn. In some newborn babies the respiratory function is depressed and the baby finds it difficult to breathe. The degree of depression can be estimated by the Apgar score, a method devised by Virginia Apgar, an American paediatrician. Five clinical signs

are looked for and are recorded at 1 minute and 5 minutes after birth. The two most important signs are the heart rate and the ability of the baby to breathe (respiratory effort). A total score of 7 or more means the baby is well and should cause no anxiety. A score of 0 to 3 indicates severe respiratory depression and tells the doctor that urgent measures need to be taken in order to resuscitate the baby.

Sign	Score 0	Score 1	Score 2
1. Colour	Blue; pale	Body pink; extremities blue	Completely pink
2. Respiratory effort	Absent	Weak cry; hypoventilation	Good; strong cry
3. Muscle tone	Limp	Some flexion of extremities	Active motion; extremities well flexed
4. Reflex irritability (response to stimulation of sole of foot)	No response	Grimace	Cry
5. Heart rate	Absent	Slow (below 100)	Fast (over 100)

Aphrodisiacs

Aphrodisiacs, or erotic stimulants, have been known since about 2000 BC, when recipes for making 'love potions' were inscribed in an Egyptian papyrus. Since that time a considerable and bizarre variety of substances have been claimed to be useful either to improve the waning sexual powers of men or to arouse the lusts of women. Most of the literature about aphrodisiacs is sexist. In various parts of the world today, certain substances

are prescribed as erotic stimulants, either powdered or pounded and mixed in various liquids. In East Asia, rhinoceros horn drunk in wine is considered valuable; in Africa, yohimbine, obtained from the bark of a tree, is claimed to increase a man's sexual power; in the Caribbean, cantharides (Spanish fly), which irritates the lining of the urinary tract, is used; in Europe, oysters and alcohol, particularly champagne, are still thought to arouse women and heighten men's sexuality. Alcohol is thought to be an aphrodisiac but is a sedative. In small quantities it makes a person less inhibited, socially and sexually, but in larger amounts leads to sleep. There is no substance which has aphrodisiac powers, unless the person taking it believes in it, when it may work.

Artificial Insemination by Donor (AID)

When a couple are found to be unable to have children because the man has no sperm in his ejaculate, or the quality of the sperm is very poor, there are three possible choices open to them. The first is to accept the situation that they will not have a child. The second is to place their names with an adoption agency. The third is for the woman to be inseminated with sperm provided by an unknown donor. This is known as Artificial Insemination by Donor (AID). As adoption is increasingly difficult to arrange because fewer babies are available, many couples now choose this course. AID services can be obtained in many hospitals and clinics in most developed countries.

The procedure is relatively simple. The time of the woman's *ovulation is determined either by measuring hormones in her blood over a period of 3 to 4 days, or by checking the quantity and character of the secretions of her cervix, or by scrutinizing a temperature chart which she has made. At ovulation time the donated semen is injected into the cervix (and sometimes into the area around the cervix) by a special syringe. The woman lies on her back for about 20 minutes with her knees bent. The insemination may be repeated the following day.

Fresh donor semen may be used but often this is difficult to arrange and increasingly frozen semen is being used. The donor's semen is placed in plastic 'straws' immediately after ejaculation (each 'straw' contains 0.5 ml) and frozen in liquid nitrogen. It can be kept for about 12 months, and used when required. Great care is taken in the selection of donors. A full medical and surgical history is obtained, the family history is reviewed to exclude familial diseases, and the donor's blood is tested to exclude venereal disease and hepatitis. A specimen of his semen is checked to make sure it is of good quality.

The results from AID show that over a 6-month period about 60 per cent of women achieve a pregnancy, and there is little difference in the result whether fresh or frozen semen is used.

B

Baby sling

In most developing countries small babies are carried around by their mothers in a sling (a *mei-tai*). The baby responds to the closeness of his mother and can feed on demand, while the mother is able to work in the house or in the fields. Psychologists believe that babies who are looked after in this way obtain more sensations than babies left in cots, where vision is limited by the side of the cot or the ceiling, and are generally happier and more placid. Mothers in developed countries are now increasingly beginning to use baby slings and are finding that the views of the experts are largely true.

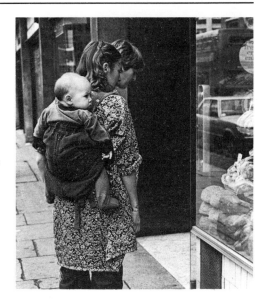

Bad breath

Bad breath is usually due to food material decaying in the mouth, or to tobacco or alcohol. The treatment is quite simply to rinse out your mouth with water and to brush your teeth. If you choose to use one of the widely advertised mouth-washes, you may do so, but there is no evidence that they are better than plain water. In some cases bad breath is due to a head cold or to a sinus infection. Persistent bad breath is usually caused by dental decay, and a dentist should be consulted.

Barr bodies

All the cells of a woman's body contain 46 *chromosomes, including two large sex chromosomes called X chromosomes. The cells of a man's body also have 46 chromosomes, including two sex chromosomes, one large X chromosome and one small Y chromosome. A woman therefore has more genetic material. In order to provide a balance in genetic material, one of the X chromosomes in each female cell becomes tightly coiled and migrates to the edge of the nucleus inside the cell. This chromosome is called a Barr body and can be seen through a microscope. If a baby has ambiguous genitals (*adrenogenital syndrome), a swab is taken from inside its cheek and a smear of the cells made on a slide; the slide is then stained with a special dye. One hundred cells are examined, and if more than 25 of the cells show Barr bodies then the baby is female.

Bartholin's abscess/cyst

*Bartholin's glands are two pea-sized organs, located one on each side of the lower part of the entrance to the vagina. A narrow canal (duct), which opens just below the hymen, connects each gland to the vagina. In some cases bacteria may enter the gland through the duct, causing infection and swelling. This leads to a blockage of the duct, and the gland fills with pus. The surrounding tissues are affected and a painful swelling develops; this is known as a *Bartholin's abscess*. In other cases the duct becomes blocked by over-growth of its cells and the fluid secreted by the gland is unable to escape. Over a period of time this leads to the development of a *Bartholin's cyst*.

A Batholin's abscess is treated by means of antibiotics and by incising the abscess and leaving a drain in the cavity for a few days. In some cases the edges of the incision are stitched to the skin, so that the gland forms an open pouch (like the pouch of a female kangaroo, hence the name which is given to the operation – marsupialization). Marsupialization is also the usual treatment for a Bartholin's cyst.

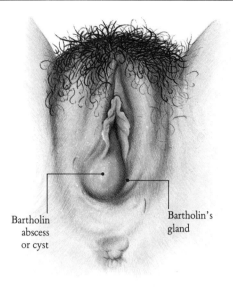

Bartholin's abscess is caused by bacteria infecting the Bartholin's glands. A cyst is caused when the ducts from the glands are blocked

Beta–agonists

Beta-agonist drugs have several uses in medicine. For example, salbutamol (Ventolin) is effective in the treatment of asthma, and both salbutamol and ritodrine (Yutopar) are used to suppress uterine activity in some cases of premature labour. Depending on the dose required, the drugs may cause side-effects such as palpitations, flushing, a rapid heart rate, and headaches. They should not be used in pregnancy if the woman has a high blood pressure or is diabetic. Usually the drug is given to a patient in the first instance as an intravenous infusion in order to suppress ★premature labour, and the dose can be continued as tablets taken by mouth after about 24 hours. The value of salbutamol and ritodrine in preventing premature labour is still under study.

Birth canal

During ★childbirth the cervix opens progressively until it disappears. When this has occurred the first stage of labour is completed. The uterus containing the fetus and the vagina form a curved tube through which the fetus has to pass to be born. This is the birth canal. The head descends downwards and backwards in a straight line until it reaches the middle of the pelvis, then its direction changes to move downwards and forwards.

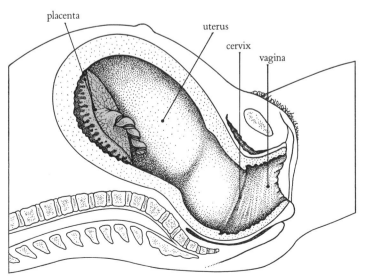

The birth canal, as shown, at the end of the first stage of labour with the cervix open

Birth Centres

Hospitals have begun to recognize the need to provide facilities for those couples who wish to have 'family-centred childbirth', which means that the woman wishes to give birth in an environment which is as similar to that in her own home as possible. She wants her partner, and perhaps her other children, to share the experience with her, as she believes childbirth to be a significant event in the life of the family. She wants to be able to cuddle her baby immediately after birth so that the process of ★bonding between her and the baby is begun as soon as possible. She wants her baby to remain with her so that she can learn about it and can breast-feed it when it wants food.

To meet these expectations, a number of hospitals have established Birth Centres. These are furnished like a bedroom with a double bed, curtains, and easy chairs. Any equipment needed for childbirth is kept discreetly hidden. The woman who chooses a Birth Centre has the satisfaction of knowing that she is giving birth in as 'natural' a way as possible, but also that if anything goes wrong – such as a change in the rate of the baby's heart, indicating that it may be at risk, or prolapse of the umbilical cord, or haemorrhage – expert medical help and special equipment are available within seconds. It can be said that a Birth Centre provides all the advantages of home birth without its possible dangers.

In the Birth Centre, the expectant mother may be cared for by a trained nurse-midwife or may choose a doctor to help her give birth. In either case the medical attendant involves the family in the experience of labour and childbirth, but has the necessary knowledge and skill so that action can be taken if intervention is needed to rescue the baby.

Studies have shown that those women who choose to give birth in a Birth Centre require fewer drugs, have fewer operative deliveries, and have fewer inductions of labour than women who choose other facilities. About 15 per cent of women who choose to give birth in a Birth Centre have to be transferred to a standard delivery unit for various reasons.

Birth injuries

As a result of improved obstetric care and skilled attention, very few babies are injured during childbirth. Occasionally the baby develops a ★cephalhaematoma and, rarely, a fractured skull. If the birth is difficult, requiring forceps, a few babies have paralysis of the facial nerve, which responds completely, without treatment, in 2 or 3 weeks. After a difficult ★breech delivery, occasionally a baby develops temporary paralysis of one of its arms. The arm is put in a splint for a while, and recovery is good.

Bisexuality

A bisexual person is attracted to members of both sexes and obtains sexual and emotional fulfilment with males and females. It is not a new condition: Alexander the Great and Julius Caesar were bisexual. Bisexuality is another variant in patterns of sexual behaviour, as are heterosexuality and homosexuality. Its origins are unknown, but it is not considered to be due to poor parenting. Occasionally, bisexuality represents a transitional stage between a heterosexual and a homosexual orientation, but there are relatively few people in this stage. Most bisexuals have a relationship with a person of one sex, and when this ends they form a new relationship with a person of the other sex; a few bisexuals have simultaneous bisexual relationships – one with a man and one with a woman. Bisexual people do not usually discover their bisexuality until their late twenties, but this varies considerably between individuals. Because of society's disapproval of homosexual relationships, a bisexual person may feel guilty, depressed, or alienated. In such cases the opportunity to talk with a sensitive, qualified therapist or counsellor may do a great deal to alleviate these feelings. Help may also be required if one partner in a permanent heterosexual relationship admits to being bisexual, but the need is not necessarily greater than if one partner of a heterosexual relationship has an affair. Bisexuals have a clear idea of their sexual orientation; they are not ambiguous (or, in colloquial terms, AC/DC), nor are they homosexuals protecting their identity.

Bleeding in late pregnancy

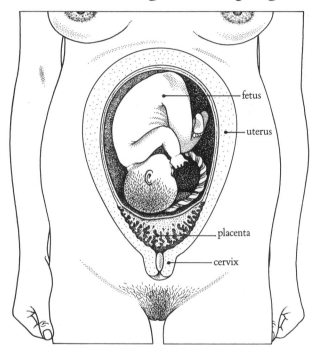

Placenta praevia showing the placenta covering the opening of the cervix

Bleeding after the 20th week of pregnancy is referred to as antepartum haemorrhage. It occurs in about 3 per cent of pregnancies, usually during the last 10 weeks. Two distinct clinical forms of antepartum haemorrhage exist. In the first form, called 'placenta praevia', the ★placenta lies in part or wholly in front of the fetus, effectively filling the lower part of the uterus. In the second form, called 'abruptio placentae' or 'accidental haemorrhage', the placenta is implanted normally in the upper part of the uterus but part of it separates from its attachment to the lining of the uterus.

Placenta praevia occurs once in every 200 pregnancies and is more common if the woman has been pregnant before. Typically, the bleeding is painless, seems to have no cause, and tends to recur. The diagnosis is made by examining the woman's abdomen, and is confirmed by taking an ★ultrasound picture. If the first bleed occurs before the 37th week of pregnancy, the woman has to remain in hospital as a further unexpected episode of bleeding may occur and be heavy. She need not stay in bed. If the condition occurs after the 37th week of pregnancy, the baby is usually delivered within a few hours of the bleeding.

In minor forms of placenta praevia, where the placenta only 'dips' into the lower part of the uterus, the ★waters may be broken to start labour and vaginal delivery may be expected. In most cases the placenta occupies more or all of the lower part of the uterus, so that ★Caesarean section is the safest treatment for both mother and baby.

Abruptio placentae occurs in about 2 per cent of pregnancies. The separation of the placenta may only affect a small part of its surface. The pregnancy can continue in this case until the normal time of delivery. If a greater area of the placenta separates from the lining, the uterus may become tender, and the woman very ill. These cases constitute obstetric emergencies, but only occur rarely. The woman is given blood transfusions, and the waters are usually broken to induce labour, if it is not in progress already. In mild cases the separation of the placenta causes no increased danger to the baby, but in severe cases the baby is often dead in the uterus before any action can be taken to save it.

Bloating, periodic

A number of women over the age of 30 find that periodically they wake up with puffy hands and face. As the day goes on, the woman may find her belly becomes distended, and she feels bloated and uncomfortable. By evening her ankles are swollen and she has gained more than 1.5 kg in weight as a result of retained fluid. The attack may last for one or more days, after which the symptoms disappear, only to recur again unexpectedly. During an attack the woman may become irritable and possibly depressed, and may also suffer from constipation. Some women find that attacks occur in the week before menstruation, or in hot weather.

Periodic bloating is due to a leak of fluid from the circulation into the tissues but it is not known why this occurs – hence its correct name 'idiopathic oedema'. Smoking aggravates the condition, so it is advisable to stop; *diuretics given at intervals may help, and taking bran can alleviate constipation.

Blood pressure

The pressure of blood in the arteries varies. When the heart beats, forcing blood into the arteries, the pressure rises (this is called the systolic pressure); between heart beats, the pressure falls (the diastolic pressure). Blood pressure is measured with an instrument called a sphygmomanometer; this consists of an inflatable cuff which is placed around the upper arm and blown up. When the pressure in the cuff exceeds the diastolic blood pressure, a thumping noise can be heard by means of a stethoscope placed over the artery in the bend of the elbow. When the pressure in the cuff exceeds that of the systolic blood pressure, the thumps cease.

Blood pressure varies during the day; anxiety increases it, tranquillity reduces it. Among people in Western countries increasing age and increasing weight lead to an increase in the blood pressure, especially in the diastolic blood pressure. In pregnancy, about 7 per cent of women experience a rise in blood pressure (*pre-eclampsia) but in nearly every case this subsides to within the normal range after childbirth.

High blood pressure (or *hypertension*), which usually occurs in later life, after the age of 45, carries potential dangers unless treated. People with high blood pressure may have a stroke, develop heart failure or kidney damage, or haemorrhage into the retina of the eye. These serious conditions can be diminished if every person aged 35 and over who visits a doctor, for whatever reason, has his or her blood pressure checked once a year. If the blood pressure is found to be high, then the reading is checked again to make sure that the rise was not due to emotional causes. If it is confirmed that the person has hypertension then treatment is started. This may include restriction of salt in the diet; reduction of weight (if the person is obese); stopping smoking; taking more exercise; learning relaxation; and the prescription of anti-hypertensive drugs.

Low blood pressure is often blamed for fatigue, lassitude fainting, and other conditions. It is unlikely that low blood pressure is the cause of any medical problem unless it results from injury, haemorrhage, or shock.

Body-image

In present-day Western society the prevalent cultural fashion is for young women to be thin and athletic. It is thought that to be thin is to be beautiful. During the four years before *puberty, as marked by the first menstrual period, a spurt of growth occurs. To meet the energy needs of this rapid time of growth, girls tend to eat more, and a habit of eating well develops. The growth spurt slows down in the year after menstruation has been established, and less energy is required by the body, so that weight will increase if the girl continues to eat the same amount of food. The gangly look of early adolescence is replaced by the 'puppy fat' of mid-adolescence. Unless the girl reduces her food intake, she may see herself as being fatter than is fashionable. This induces her to diet to lose weight, and often to alternate dieting with episodes of over-eating. Studies in several countries show that over 60 per cent of adolescent women diet intermittently to improve their 'body-image' and to feel 'good' about their shape. Thirty per cent of adolescents admit to experiencing binge-eating (★bulimia) at some time. In addition, a small number of young women use potentially dangerous methods of losing weight, such as self-induced vomiting, or excessive use of laxatives, slimming tablets, or diuretics. Other women become obsessed with taking exercise in order to keep a good body-image. In most cases the behaviours are under control but in some instances a few women may become binge-eaters; others, however, so rigidly restrict their food intake that they may become extremely thin or develop ★anorexia nervosa.

Body odour

Body odour is caused by the modification of sweat by bacteria, producing chemicals which smell. Sweating occurs during hot weather, more particularly if tight-fitting clothes or synthetic fabrics are worn, and in response to anxiety, fear, or stress. The parts of the body where sweating usually occurs are in the armpits, under the breasts, in the groin, and in the case of sweating induced by stress, on the palms, the feet, and the face.

In most cases, deodorants will control the odour of sweat, but stress-induced sweating may need other measures. One treatment is to apply a substance of aluminium chloride hexahydrate (20 per cent in alcohol) to the armpits, especially at night.

Bondage

Some people feel a psychological need during love-play to be demonstrably dominant, making the sex partner into a submissive postulant. This can be achieved by verbal games or, more often, by sex games involving fantasy. In the fantasy one partner imposes his or her will on the other, making the person a slave, who may be chastised or 'tortured' at will. This is called erotic bondage. Men who are passive and unassertive in life, and in love-making, may seek erotic bondage as it gives them the opportunity to play out their fantasy of being aggressive and dominant. Sex shops have a large variety of equipment for bondage – ropes, belts, lacing, wrist and body straps, gags, chains, face-masks; leather is a preferred material. The fantasy games take various forms but in each case the 'victim' is eventually expected to accept being bound by the dominant partner and to submit to 'punishments' which have been jointly agreed.

There are obvious dangers in the techniques of erotic bondage and no person should allow another to practise these techniques unless both partners are confident that certain rules will be observed. These are that bondage must be with the consent of both partners; both must be completely sober; a person who is tied up must never be left alone; when a previously agreed signal is given, the 'victim' must be immediately released from all restraints; nothing must be placed around the neck, or the breathing restricted in any way; any knots or leather clasps which are used must be easily unfastened.

Bonding

Bonding is the process which usually begins in the first hours after birth and continues over the following days or weeks so that a stable emotional link and an affectionate attachment are formed between a mother and her baby (and, by extension, between father and baby).

Bonding depends on a number of sequential events, all of which are desirable but none essential. The first is that the pregnancy is planned and that the birth of the baby is anticipated with pleasure. In pregnancy, *quickening confirms that the fetus has an identity. Bonding is encouraged if childbirth takes place in a pleasant environment, and if the medical and nursing attendants are warm, supportive, and talk with the expectant mother. Bonding is further encouraged if, immediately after the baby has been born, the parents are given the opportunity to touch, feel, and smell the baby. The care of the newborn and young baby by his mother adds to the emotional link.

The process of bonding is facilitated by physical contact between the parent (usually the mother) and the baby – by skin-to-skin contact, by suckling, by looking at the baby,

by talking to the baby, and by fondling him. It is the beginning of the development of *mother-love.

Some paediatricians believe that if parents are denied the opportunity to see their baby, to touch and care for him (or at least to participate in his care) in the first two weeks of life, then a number of problems may arise later. These can include less affectionate behaviour in the mother and a reduction in the duration of breast-feeding.

Whether the supposed benefits of bonding are real or not, it is natural for a mother and her partner to want to be left together with their healthy baby immediately after he has been born, to celebrate his birth, to explore his body, and to show the baby, and each other, the love and affection which exists between them. This can be arranged easily if the birth has been normal or if a *forceps delivery has been necessary. It can also be arranged if the woman has needed a *Caesarean section, as the operation can now take place under *epidural anaesthesia and the father can be present. Even if the baby requires intensive care, the parents can visit him and initiate the bonding process.

Braxton-Hicks contractions

The uterus contracts at intervals of 15 to 30 minutes throughout the reproductive years. In pregnancy the contractions become stronger and more obvious, particularly in the last 10 weeks. Although they are painless, they are noticed by the expectant mother as a definite hardening of the uterus, which lasts about 30 seconds.

The contractions were first reported by an English doctor called John Braxton-Hicks in

1872, and have been given his name. In contradistinction to the contractions of labour, Braxton-Hicks contractions do not lead to the opening of the cervix. However, they do lead to an alternating flow of blood into the uterus which helps to nourish the fetus. Braxton-Hicks contractions may also induce the fetus to move, so causing it to use its muscles, which is naturally beneficial to its development.

Breast anatomy

The breasts are unique organs as they not only fulfil a vitally important function in providing the most appropriate food for a baby, but they also play a powerful erotic role. Until *puberty the breasts are small,

but as a result of the stimulating effects of the female sex hormones they begin to develop.

The anatomy of the breast has been graphically described as 'a forest of ten or twenty trees all intimately bound together by

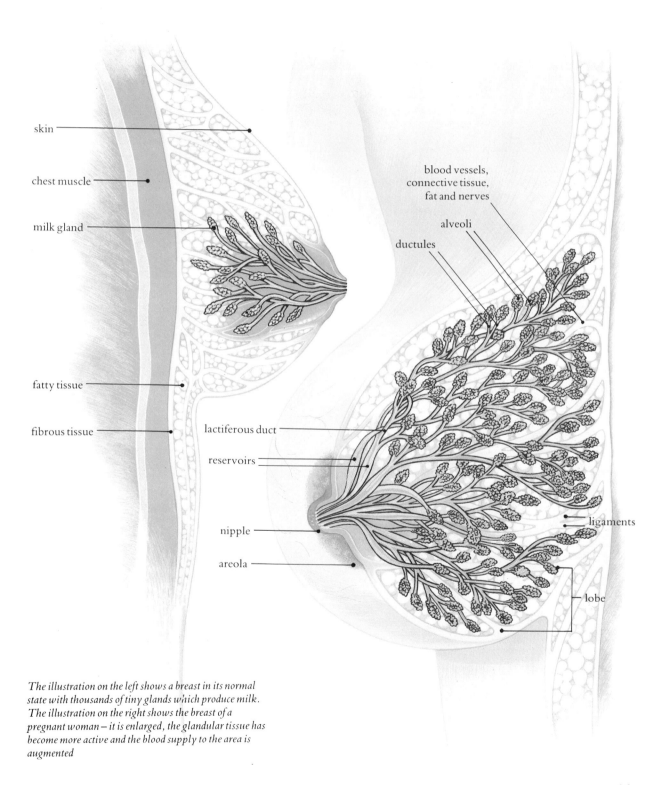

skin

chest muscle

milk gland

blood vessels,
connective tissue,
fat and nerves

alveoli

ductules

fatty tissue

fibrous tissue

lactiferous duct

reservoirs

ligaments

nipple

areola

lobe

*The illustration on the left shows a breast in its normal
state with thousands of tiny glands which produce milk.
The illustration on the right shows the breast of a
pregnant woman – it is enlarged, the glandular tissue has
become more active and the blood supply to the area is
augmented*

interweaving vines and vegetation'. The 'trees' are the ten to twenty hollow milk ducts which develop in each breast. Each *milk duct* opens into the nipple and extends through the breast tissues, branching again and again as smaller ductules, to end deep in the breast, in the milk-secreting sacs called *alveoli*, hollow balls of cells surrounded by tiny muscles. Each milk (or lactiferous) duct system forms a breast *lobe*, which is partially separated from the other lobes by condensations of tissue, which form ligaments in the substance of the breast. The *ligaments* stretch from the fibrous tissue which lies behind the breasts almost to the skin which covers it, and help to support the breast. As a woman grows older, the ligaments tend to lose their elasticity, with the result that the breasts may become less firm and sag. The lobes divide into smaller lobes (lobules), which are separated from each other by fat through which

blood vessels pass (the 'interweaving vines and vegetation'). In turn each lobe is made up of between 10 and 100 milk-producing alveoli.

The size and shape of the breasts do not depend on the number of lobes and lobules, but on the amount of fat deposited in and around them, and the quality of the ligaments within the breast. They vary in size during the menstrual cycle, enlarging in the days before the menstrual period by between 8 and 40 per cent.

Surrounding the *nipple* is a disc of thin skin called the *areola*. In the substance of the nipple as well as the outlet of the ducts there are tiny muscles which contract when stimulated either by cold or by touch, to make the nipple erect. The sensitivity of the nipple to touch varies between individual women but is greatest during the middle part of the menstrual cycle.

Breast cancer

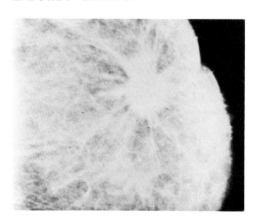

Breast cancer can be detected by mammography when an X-ray photograph is taken using equipment that gives films of high-quality definition enabling easier diagnosis of lumps or tumours. This mammogram shows a lump which proved to be a cancer

It has been estimated that one in 25 of all female children born in the United Kingdom will develop breast cancer at some time in her life, usually after the age of 50. Women who have given birth to a baby before the age of 25 have half the risk of developing the disease, while women with a close relative who

has had breast cancer have twice the risk. Breast cancer is not caused by a blow to the breast, by bruising or bites, or by a virus.

It is a matter of concern that the death rate from breast cancer has not decreased since 1910, in spite of a variety of new treatments. The reason for this is that unless the disease is detected early, unnoticed spread to distant organs is likely to have occurred, and breast surgery on its own, however radical, is unlikely to influence the death rate.

These facts have led to a different approach to breast cancer. The first new initiative is that women are encouraged to carry out a regular ★self-examination of their breasts, and from the age of 40 to have an annual breast check made by a doctor. The doctor may include a ★mammogram as part of the examination, so that any cancer is detected at an early stage. The second change is that increasing numbers of surgeons are abandoning the extensive breast surgery which women feared and which resulted in a deformity. It is becoming increasingly common to remove the affected breast and 'samples' from the lymph nodes in the armpit. The nodes are examined by a pathologist to see if they contain cancer cells. If they do not, then the outlook for the woman is very good, but if they do, further treatment using X-rays (radiotherapy) or drugs (*chemotherapy) is required.

Some surgeons are more conservative in certain cases of breast cancer and preserve most of the breast by performing what is rather inelegantly called a 'lumpectomy'. In this operation, the area containing the cancer is removed together with a surrounding area of healthy tissue, and the shape of the breast is restored as far as possible. If a recurrence of cancer occurs in the breast area then radio-

therapy is thought to be the most appropriate treatment. The treatment of breast cancer remains controversial but it is hoped that these changes in attitude and approach will reduce the death rate.

Each woman who is diagnosed as having breast cancer is entitled to discuss with her doctor the treatment he intends to use and the help she will be given to adjust to the loss of her breast. She should also be advised of those measures (such as a breast shape or prosthesis) which will help her to retain her sense of femininity after the emotional trauma of the operation. (See *Mastectomy.)

Breast enlargement

In this 'mammarized world' (to quote an American plastic surgeon) a woman may think that her breasts are unfashionably small. If she sees her breasts as unattractive she may also feel insecure, inadequate, and depressed, and she may wish to have bigger breasts which will be more sexually attractive. The size of the breasts cannot be increased by exercises, although by improving her general posture a woman may make her breasts appear more prominent. Nor do ointments rubbed into the breasts increase their size significantly, although ointments which contain oestrogen may cause a slight increase. Small-breasted women may observe that their breasts become slightly larger when taking the contraceptive *pill.

The only way in which the size of the breasts can be increased to any considerable degree is by what plastic surgeons call 'augmentation mammoplasty'. The surgeon makes a small incision around the edge of the areola (the area surrounding the nipple) and then by 'tunnelling' between the skin and the breast tissue he reaches the space behind the breast and the underlying muscle. Alternatively, he may reach the space by making a curved incision in the fold below the breast. He introduces a shaped silicone sac (of a size decided between the woman and the surgeon) which is filled with a plastic jelly. The sac is soft and pliable and by pushing the breast tissue forward gives the breast the new, enlarged shape the woman desires.

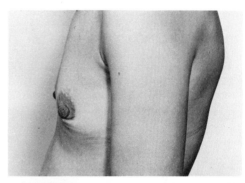

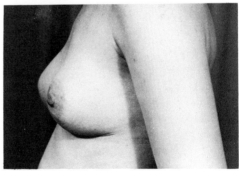

Once the scars have healed, they fade and in 6 to 9 months the incisions are barely visible. Most women are delighted with the results but in a few cases the body reacts to the silicone implant and produces thick fibrous tissue which contracts around the implant, giving it a firm texture and an unnatural shape. This can be corrected by means of surgery.

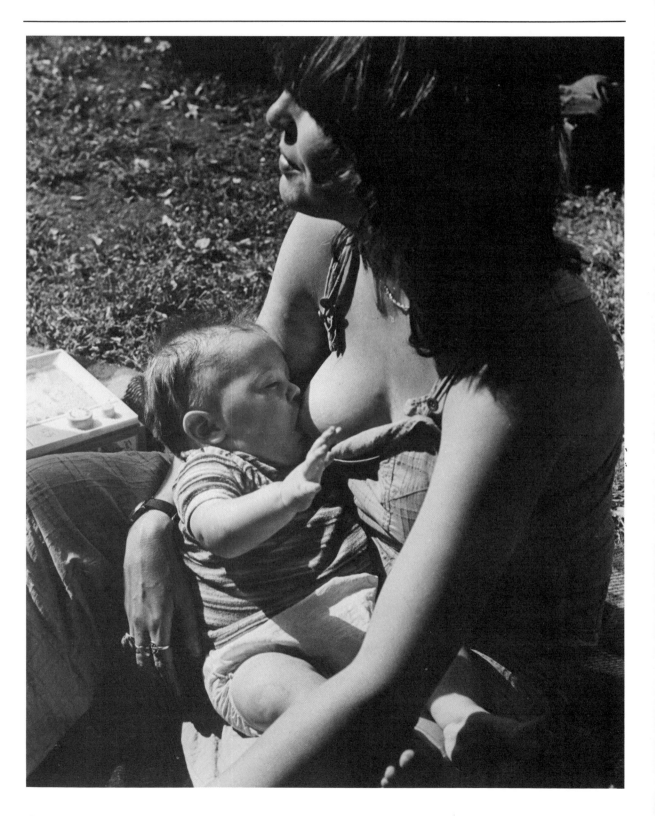

Breast-feeding

Until about a hundred years ago most women breast-fed their babies or, if they were rich, employed a 'wet nurse'. With the development of formula feeds based on cow's milk, bottle-feeding became fashionable. By the 1950s, fewer than one-quarter of mothers in Britain and the United States chose to breast-feed, and at least half of them stopped breast-feeding within 3 months. Since the mid-1970s there has been a modest return to breast-feeding, particularly among middle-class women.

Breast-feeding, which supplies human milk, has several advantages. For the mother, breast-feeding is generally less time-consuming than bottle-feeding, it increases the interaction between mother and baby, and it has a pleasurable erotic effect on many mothers.

The benefits of breast-feeding as far as the baby is concerned are considerable. Breast milk is the most appropriate, nutritionally balanced, 'protective' food for the baby's growth and development. Breast milk contains anti-infective substances (absent in cow's or formula milk) which protect the baby against gastrointestinal and respiratory infections. Breast-feeding, provided no supplementary feeds of formula milk are given, reduces the likelihood that the baby will develop allergic eczema or asthma.

Babies are individuals and require to be fed as individuals, preferably by *demand feeding. The amount of breast milk taken each feed varies considerably but usually a balance of supply and demand is reached quickly. Most babies need no other food than breast milk for the first 4 to 6 months of their life and most mothers, provided they are completely relaxed and confident about their ability to breast-feed, can supply all the milk the baby needs.

Breast-feeding has been called a 'confidence trick': the more confident the mother, the more likely she is to initiate and maintain breast-feeding. Her confidence is increased if she has someone to whom she can talk when she is anxious. This may be her doctor, a health worker, or one of the organizations which help breast-feeding mothers such as the La Leche League International in the United States, the Nursing Mothers Association in Australia, or the National Childbirth Trust in the United Kingdom.

Breast infection

Most breast infections occur during breast-feeding, when bacteria enter the breast through a fissure or 'crack' in the nipple; this may result in a 'caked breast' or mastitis. In a few cases, one of the tiny glands (Montgomery's tubercles) in the areola surrounding the nipple may be infected. A small lump appears, which contains pus. Antibiotics usually clear it up, but occasionally it has to be incised (lanced).

The cause of *caked breast* (more properly called 'intermammary mastitis') is not certain, but it is probably due to infection which leads to swelling of a lobe of the breast. The swelling blocks the duct draining the lobe, and the result is a tender area in the breast with a patch of reddened skin. The woman feels feverish, aches all over, and has a raised temperature. In the early stages before it has developed fully, 'caked breast' may be prevented by feeding the baby often, and by expressing all the remaining milk from the breast by hand after each feed. Massaging the breast and the application of hot and cold towels are also said to help. If the condition persists, however, then the woman will have developed mastitis.

Mastitis affects about 2 per cent of breast-feeding mothers and can be painful. The woman has a tense, tender area in her breast, and pus may form in it. She feels generally unwell and has a raised temperature. If mastitis is treated in its early stages then it may be possible to prevent a breast abscess from developing. There are two principles involved in treatment. The first is that the woman should empty her breast regularly by frequently feeding the baby. This may cause discomfort and she may wish to take aspirin or some other analgesic about half an hour before feeding. The second principle is that large doses of penicillin (usually Flucloxacillin) should be given by mouth as early as possible to prevent the formation of an abscess.

Breast abscess occurs in about 7 per cent of women who have mastitis. After treatment with antibiotics, the abscess has to be incised under anaesthesia. The mother should not feed the baby from the affected breast until healing is complete but she can feed from the other breast.

Breast lumps

It is quite common for women to notice that in the two weeks or so before menstruation their breasts become bigger and develop tender areas of knobbly lumps, rather like thick, tangled string, usually in the upper and outer part of each breast. Once menstruation starts the tenderness goes and the lumps disappear. This condition is part of the *premenstrual syndrome.

Some women over the age of 30 develop a second form of breast lumpiness which is an exaggeration of the type which occurs before menstruation. Unlike the first type, the lumpiness may persist throughout the menstrual cycle. It is believed to be due to an excessive sensitivity to the sex hormones which leads to increased growth of the breast tissues – the 'milk tree'. In some cases the cells which form the 'tree' grow inwards and block one of the ducts, so that a cyst or several cysts form. The lumpiness can be quite marked and a tender area can occur, causing discomfort which varies in intensity from day to day.

The two conditions overlap and have a variety of names, the most common being 'benign breast disease', to emphasize that the condition is not a cancer. Many women tolerate the discomfort, once they have been reassured that they do not have breast cancer. Others require medication, but none is particularly satisfactory. Newer drugs such as *bromocriptine, *danazol, and dydrogesterone may help, and their place and usefulness will be defined more clearly in the future.

Other women, when they examine their breasts following a menstrual period, discover a lump or a lumpy area. These lumps are rather common, and one woman in 5 will detect a lump or a lumpy area at some time during her life. Her immediate thought is that she has *breast cancer, but 4 out of every 5 lumps are not due to cancer. However, all breast lumps should be examined by a doctor.

In young women, the most common lump is called a fibroadenoma. The lump is smooth, firm, and painless and it seems to move under the woman's probing fingers, which has led to it being called a 'breast mouse'. Although it is not a cancer the woman should nevertheless see a doctor. In many cases he will advise that the lump be removed as 'breast mice' often continue to grow.

Breast lumps or lumpy areas require investigation and a doctor should be consulted. He will examine the breast and may suggest a *mammogram or an *ultrasound picture to help him in his diagnosis. After this he may suggest that the lump be examined by inserting a narrow needle through the tissues of the breast, to take a sample of the lump or, if it is a cyst, to empty it. Sometimes the whole lump may have to be removed so that it can be examined in the laboratory. The operation is a minor one, and the woman need only remain in hospital for a day or two.

Eighty per cent of breast lumps are not cancerous, but many women who detect a lump in their breasts delay seeking medical advice, often for more than 3 months. The reasons for the delay are varied but a common reason is that the woman fears the lump will be a cancer, which she believes erroneously to be painful and incurable. Today, with better methods of early detection and new methods of treatment, women with *early* cancer have an 80 per cent chance of being cured.

Breast milk

Composition of human milk and cow's milk

Biochemical Substance	Human Milk	Cow's Milk
Water per 100ml	87.1	87.3
Total solids g/100ml		
Protein	0.9	3.3
Casein % of total	20	82
Whey % of total	80	18
Fat	4.5	3.7
Milk sugar (lactose)	6.8	4.8
Minerals mg/100ml		
Calcium mg	34	125
Phosphorus mg	14	96
Sodium mmol/litre	7	25
Vitamins		
Vitamin A μg	54	30
Vitamin B_1 μg	15	37
Vitamin B_2 μg	38	180
Vitamin B_6 μg	13	46
Vitamin C mg μg	43	11
Energy provided kcal/100ml	75	69

Breast milk is the most appropriate, nutritionally balanced, 'protective' food for the human baby in the first 6 months of his life, or longer. Cow's milk, however modified, can never be as good as breast milk, although if it is prepared in accordance with the recommendations of the manufacturer, using sterilized bottles and teats, it is a safe and satisfactory way of feeding a baby. Breast milk and cow's milk are compared in the table opposite.

Breast milk is superior to cow's milk as a food for human infants for the following reasons:

Its protein consists of 80 per cent whey which is easily digested and contains protective substances which prevent infection.

The curd which is formed by the action of enzymes in the stomach on the casein protein is soft and frothy, which enables the baby to absorb more protein.

Its fat content is better balanced and more easily digested.

Its sugar content (lactose) is higher, which provides energy and aids in the absorption of calcium from the milk.

Although its calcium content is lower, the calcium is more readily absorbed.

Breast reduction

A few young women develop breasts which so exceed the fashionable size or sag to such an extent that the woman feels that she is an object of ridicule. Occasionally one breast grows abnormally larger than the other. To some extent large breasts are associated with obesity, and weight reduction by dieting will reduce their size. This is a particular problem among older women aged between 35 and 55 who are obese. The size of her breasts may embarrass the woman, or cause her physical pain in her back or neck as the heavy breasts sag, or the straps of her bra create deep grooves over her shoulder-bones. The skin in the fold below the breasts may become moist and itchy rashes may occur. If the woman enjoys playing active sports, such as tennis, the weight of her breasts may cause her pain.

Plastic surgeons have now developed techniques which enable the removal of large quantities of fatty tissue from the breasts to restore their shape ('reduction mammoplasty'). This is done in such a way that the scars are more or less concealed. In the first 3 to 6 months after surgery the scars are red, but after one year they have usually faded and are hardly noticeable.

Over 90 per cent of women who have reduction mammoplasty are well satisfied with the size and shape of their new breasts, but in the remaining cases there are problems of scar healing. There is also usually a loss of sensation in the nipples, which is a matter of concern to those women who are erotically aroused by having their nipples stimulated.

If a woman decides to have a breast reduction, she should look for a skilled plastic surgeon who performs the operation regularly. She should have a full and frank discussion with the surgeon about the benefits and the possible complications of the operation so that she is fully aware of the psychological and physical implications.

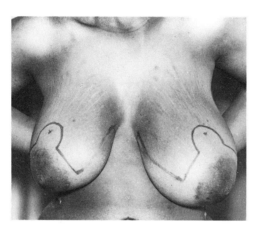 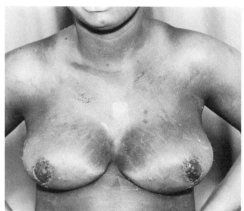

Breast self-examination

Breast self-examination (BSE) is recommended by many doctors as an important way in which a woman can detect ★breast lumps. Although 4 lumps in every 5 are not due to cancer, they can only be differentiated by medical investigation. Breast self-examination is seen as a sensible precaution for 'screening' all women. In addition, women over the age of 35 should have their breasts examined once a year by a doctor, and those over the age of 50 should have an annual ★mammogram.

The technique of breast self-examination is not difficult, but it is learned most effectively with the guidance of a health professional, who need not be a doctor. When a woman learns how to examine her own breasts, she comes to know and to appreciate their texture, and to become conscious of the thickened areas in the gland tissue which are unique and normal in her breasts. If a woman is menstruating she should examine her breasts each month in the week after her period finishes; if she has ceased to menstruate she should do the examination at the same time each month.

The examination should be done in the sequence shown opposite.

The method shown in the drawings opposite is recommended by several national cancer societies, but if it seems too complicated then you can make the following, simpler examination, which is nearly as good. Before you have a bath or shower, stand in front of a mirror, put your hands by your sides, and look at your breasts. When you are in the bath or under the shower, and your skin is wet and soapy, examine your breasts by feeling them gently all over. If you detect a lump (or an area in your breast which causes you concern), you should make an appointment to see your doctor, so that the lump can be investigated further.

A woman who does not examine her own breasts regularly should obviously have a regular medical check. If she detects a lump

You are looking at your breasts to see if the shape of either of them has changed since the last self-examination; if any part of the skin is puckered; if there is a bulge or a flattened area in either breast; or if either nipple has been drawn into the breast tissue.

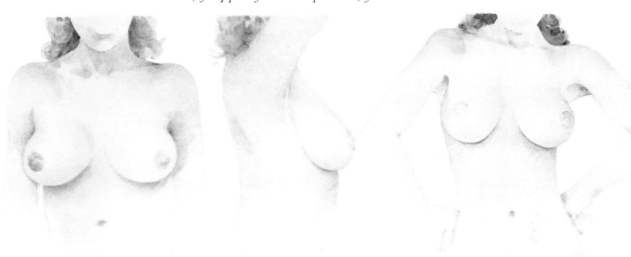

1 Stand in front of a mirror, put your hands by your sides, and look at your breasts.

2 Then raise your hands above your head and look again.

3 Now put your hands on your hips, press firmly, with the elbows forward (this stretches the pectoral muscles), and look again.

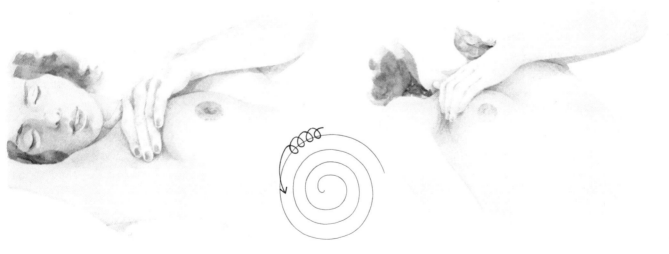

4 Next, lie down on a bed, a couch, or, if you prefer, in your bath. If you lie on a bed, put a pillow under the shoulder on the side of the breast you are going to examine. You will find it easier to examine your breast if the skin is wet and, if possible, soapy. As you examine each breast, raise the arm on that side above your head. The pillow under your shoulder, and the raised arm, spreads the breast tissue more evenly over your ribcage and makes the palpation easier. (*'Palpation' means to examine gently, using the flat of your first three fingers held together.*) Feel each breast gently and systematically with the flat of the fingers of the opposite hand. Start at the upper, outer part of the breast and work your way round, moving your fingers in small circles until you have palpated the entire breast.

5 Finally, return to the upper area, between the nipple and armpit, and palpate it again, as this is where most lumps will be found.

When you have examined one breast, repeat the same procedure on the other breast.

by chance, or because pain in her breast induces her to palpate it, she should arrange to see her doctor without delay in order that an examination can be made.

Breech baby

Up to about the 20th week of pregnancy nearly as many babies lie head up (or breech down) in the uterus as lie head down. From then on increasing numbers of babies lie head down in the uterus (cephalic position). By the 34th week only 8 per cent are in the breech position and by 40 weeks the proportion has dropped to 3 per cent. Most breech babies have their legs stretched along their bodies; some have their legs flexed at the knee and a few lie with one leg stretched downwards.

Many doctors try to manipulate a breech baby at the 34th week of pregnancy in an attempt to turn it into a head down position. However, a baby may be in a breech position when labour starts, and the more premature the labour, the higher the likelihood that the baby will lie as a breech.

Provided that the woman has a normal-sized pelvis, that her uterus contracts strongly, and that the baby is neither small (less than 2000 g) nor very large (more than 4000 g), a breech birth is no more dangerous for the mother or the baby. However, since it is difficult to estimate the size of the baby or to predict the quality of the uterine contractions, more breech babies are being born by ★Caesarean section as it is argued that this reduces the danger of cerebral damage to a small or a large baby during birth. Currently between 20 and 75 per cent of breech babies are delivered by Caesarean section, which suggests that fashion not science must influence the decision. If it is found that a woman in late pregnancy has a breech baby she may choose to discuss the method of birth with her doctor.

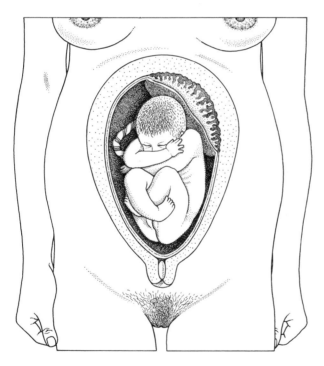

At the end of pregnancy a few babies do not take up the normal head downwards position

Bromocriptine

Recent research has shown that one woman in every 4 whose menstrual periods stop for 6 months or longer, and who is neither pregnant nor underweight, is producing excessive amounts of a hormone called ★prolactin. Prolactin is secreted by the pituitary gland and is normally controlled by a substance called dopamine which is produced in the brain. However, in certain circumstances, the pituitary gland is no longer able to control the secretion of prolactin and the level of prolactin in the blood rises. These high levels of prolactin prevent ★ovulation and cause ★amenorrhoea.

After investigation to exclude a tumour of the pituitary gland, ovulation and menstruation can be restored by giving the drug bromocriptine, which acts like dopamine to prevent the secretion of prolactin.

Bromocriptine has also been used to increase the fertility of women who have slightly raised levels of prolactin in their blood; of men who have low sperm counts and raised blood levels of prolactin; and it may help a small group of men who have erectile impotence. Bromocriptine is also used in the treatment of other conditions which are associated with raised prolactin levels in the blood.

Recently bromocriptine has been given to women who develop tender, painful breasts in the week before menstruation (★premenstrual syndrome). Improvement has been shown in about 70 per cent of women with this condition.

As prolactin is the major hormone involved in establishing and maintaining ★lactation, and as a fall in prolactin is associated with a reduction in milk secretion, bromocriptine is the preferred drug if a woman wants to avoid or to suppress lactation and breast-feeding.

Bulimia

Bulimia, or binge-eating, is an eating disorder which predominantly affects young women and is associated with a preoccupation with food and weight control. Periodically the woman goes on an eating binge, during which she eats everything she can obtain, preferring what she describes as 'bad foods', and in a day she may eat ten times her normal amount of food. The eating binges may occur very frequently and usually only last a few hours, but occasionally may last for a day or longer. It is obvious that if a woman binge-eats frequently, she will become fat rather quickly. However, most binge-eaters are of normal weight, although the condition is found among a few obese people and some women who have ★anorexia nervosa. Most binge-eaters avoid gaining weight by dieting strictly between binges, and after some years may resort to potentially dangerous behaviours to avoid weight gain. These include self-induced vomiting, eating large quantities of slimming tablets, or abusing laxatives or ★diuretics. These methods are used during each binge or between binges.

Most binge-eaters are secretive about their behaviours (at least in the early stages), and even close relatives may be unaware of their eating disorder. Eating binges occur for a number of reasons, such as unhappiness, boredom, or loneliness. Before starting an eating binge, the woman usually feels anxious and tense; during the binge, a sense of freedom or feelings of relief occur, but sometimes these pleasant sensations only occur after the woman has induced vomiting. Often, though, the woman has negative feelings about herself because of her eating behaviours, and the binge only provides a temporary relief of her tension and anxiety.

A binge-eater needs specialist help from a trained counsellor or a psychotherapist, who can help her come to terms with the disordered eating behaviours, and also give advice and support on other problems such as a sexual relationship or family difficulties which may be associated with binge-eating. Therapy is also aimed at inducing the woman to turn away from her preoccupation with food and weight.

C

Caesarean section

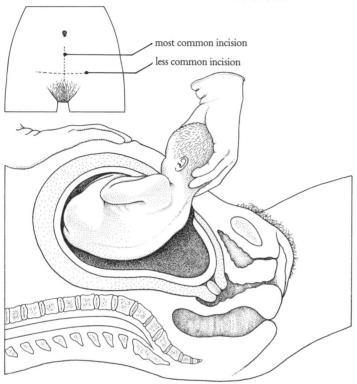

most common incision
less common incision

In a delivery by Caesarean section – which has nothing to do with Julius Caesar but comes from the word 'to cut' – the baby is removed from the intact uterus by an abdominal operation. Caesarean section is needed if the mother's pelvis is too small or her baby too big; if the placenta is lying below the baby and obstructing the cervix (*placenta praevia); or if a tumour occupies the pelvis. The operation may be advised if the woman develops high blood pressure in pregnancy; if the baby is in an abnormal position; if the umbilical cord prolapses during labour; or if the fetus becomes 'distressed' (at risk of dying because of insufficient oxygen supply via the placenta, or suffering brain damage if labour is allowed to continue to vaginal delivery). Recently, Caesarean section has been advocated if a woman starts in premature labour, and if her baby is a *breech baby. Some obstetricians advise that once a woman has been delivered by Caesarean section, every subsequent delivery should also be by Caesarean section. The operation is usually performed under general anaesthesia, but increasingly *epidural anaesthesia is being used so that the mother may hear and see her baby during his birth.

In the past fifteen years the rate of Caesarean section has risen from 4 to 8 per cent in Britain, from 8 to 15 per cent in the United States, and from 6 to 12 per cent in Australia. Fashion has played a part as the rate varies considerably between different obstetricians serving the same population. Some authorities believe that Caesarean section is performed too frequently. They agree that the operation is safe (it is still more dangerous for the mother than a 'normal' birth), but say that it is associated with and followed by more pain and discomfort than a vaginal birth. A woman who is advised by her obstetrician that she needs to have a Caesarean section is entitled to know the reason for the decision and to be told exactly what the operation will involve.

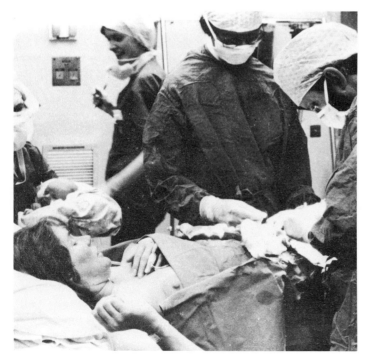

Cancer of the uterus

Although *breast cancer is the most common female cancer, about 4 per cent of women will develop cancer of the uterus at some time, usually after the age of 40. There are two main forms of uterine cancer which are distinct in their diagnosis, their progress, and their treatment. These are cancer of the uterine cervix, usually called cervical cancer, and cancer of the lining of the uterus, or endometrial cancer.

Cervical cancer This form of uterine cancer usually develops after the age of 40 and the malignant changes in the cells are preceded for between 5 and 15 years by less serious cell abnormalities. These pre-cancerous changes can be detected by means of a *cervical smear, and adequate treatment will prevent the development of cervical cancer. Unfortunately, however, not all women are prepared to have regular examinations and smear tests. In a very few cases, cancer develops with great rapidity, and it is these women in particular who are at risk. Unless it is diagnosed early, the cancer spreads from the *cervix into the tissues surrounding the uterus or into the vagina. The extent of the spread predetermines the treatment, and the earlier the cancer is detected, the higher the chance of cure. In most cancer centres, cervical cancer is treated by radium and X-rays (radiotherapy), but a few gynaecologists prefer surgery which removes the uterus, the surrounding tissues, and the upper one-third of the vagina. In terms of survival of 5 years or more, the results of the two types of treatment are similar. For this reason a woman should expect and, indeed, insist on a full and frank discussion with her doctor if cervical cancer has been diagnosed, in order that she may be involved in and understand the choice of treatment.

Endometrial cancer This type of cancer occurs rather less frequently than cervical cancer and usually affects women who have passed the *menopause. The woman is likely to be overweight, to have high blood pressure, and she may have diabetes, but not all women who develop endometrial cancer show these characteristics. These particular factors, and the known increase in the prevalence of endometrial cancer among women who have received *hormone replacement therapy for menopausal symptoms, implicate the female sex hormone *oestrogen in the development of the cancer. Endometrial cancer grows slowly and silently. Usually the first sign that a post-menopausal woman may have endometrial cancer is the appearance of a bloodstained discharge or a 'menstrual period'. Any woman who develops any vaginal bleeding after the menopause should visit a doctor urgently. The doctor will examine her and arrange for a *D and C to be carried out. About one woman in 5 who develops post-menopausal bleeding is found to have an endometrial cancer. The treatment of endometrial cancer is to remove the uterus by *hysterectomy and, if the cancer has grown deeply into the uterine tissues, to give radiation therapy following the surgery. In a few advanced, or inoperable, cases, the use of *gestagens prescribed in large doses can sometimes prolong the woman's life for a while.

Candida infections

Candida infections (candidiasis, moniliasis), commonly known as thrush, are caused by the fungus *Candida albicans* which may infect the vagina and sometimes the bowel of otherwise healthy women. Studies in several countries show that the fungus is present in the vagina of between 5 and 25 per cent of women between the ages of 15 and 50. In most women it causes no symptoms as its growth is kept in check by the other bacteria in the vagina, but occasionally it starts growing, especially if the woman is diabetic or has been treated with antibiotics. Between 2 and 4 per cent of women develop a vaginal discharge and have marked itching. Candida infections are diagnosed by taking a swab

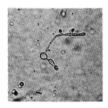

from the vagina and inoculating it into a culture medium. In 48 hours, colonies of the fungus can be seen by the naked eye.

It is important to diagnose candidiasis accurately as specific medications are available. These medications are listed in the table below.

There is little difference in the effectiveness of the available medications, and a single course of treatment will cure over 85 per cent of women. As candidiasis is sexually transmitted, the woman's partner may need treatment with a fungicidal cream applied to his penis.

Clotrimazole		**Nystatin**	
(Canesten)	1 tablet inserted in the vagina daily for 7 days	(Myostatin, Nilstat)	1 tablet inserted in the vagina twice daily for 2 weeks
Econazole		**Miconazole**	
(Ecostatin, Pervary)	1 tablet inserted in the vagina for 3 days	(Gyno-Daktarin, Monistat-7)	1 applicator full in the vagina daily for 7 days

Caput succedaneum

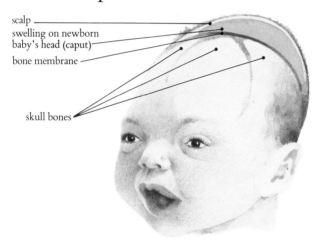

scalp
swelling on newborn baby's head (caput)
bone membrane

skull bones

Caput succedaneum is the name given to the circumscribed swelling on a newborn baby's head which occurs when there has been a tight fit between the baby's head and the ★birth canal. In most cases the swelling is only a few millimetres thick, but in a labour which has been allowed to continue for many hours (an unusual occurrence today) it may be extensive. It is due to fluid in the scalp tissues and does not involve the skull or the brain. Whatever its size, it is soft when touched. It disappears in a few days without treatment.

Caput: a swelling of the tissues of the baby's scalp which occurs during childbirth

Cardiotocography

The cardiotocograph (CTG) is a machine used for ★fetal monitoring in pregnancy. It is attached by wires to detecting devices on the mother's abdomen (or in labour on the scalp of the baby). The machine detects the baby's heart beat and electronically computes it instantaneously to the number of times it is beating each minute. Another sensor picks up the uterine contractions (if any occur). In late pregnancy the machine is started and the baby's heart beats are recorded for about half an hour. Normally the heart rate fluctuates rapidly over a small range. The mother notes when the baby kicks and records this by pressing a button. If the baby is healthy and not at risk, the heart rate will increase each time the baby moves in the uterus. If the baby is under threat, for whatever reason (see ★High-risk pregnancy), the fetal heart will not react to its movements by an increased rate, and if the threat is great the fluctuating beats will even out. In this event the doctor will discuss the problem with the woman and her partner and may decide to deliver the baby, usually by ★Caesarean section.

The cardiotocograph is also used during labour to monitor the well-being of the baby. In some hospitals, every labour is monitored, although this reduces the 'naturalness' of childbirth, and limits the mother's comfort. In other units, monitoring is carried out on all high-risk pregnancies during labour, and on other pregnancies where problems occur. Some calculations have suggested that routine monitoring saves the life of one baby in a thousand.

Caruncle, urethral

This is a small, dull red, polyp-like protrusion which appears in the entrance to the urinary tract in the ★vulva of older women. Usually it is very tender when touched or when the woman urinates. A urethral caruncle generally only occurs after the ★menopause and is thought to be a consequence of the lack of oestrogen in the tissues. A mild, painless caruncle sometimes improves if the woman places an oestrogen cream on it each day; but most caruncles are painful and need to be treated by a small surgical operation.

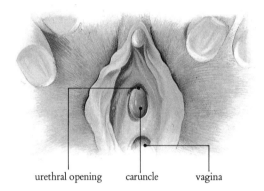

urethral opening   caruncle   vagina

Cauterization of the cervix

After childbirth, some women may have a heavy vaginal discharge which persists for a few months, although no infecting organism is found when a vaginal swab is examined in a laboratory. Physical examination shows a large ★cervical 'erosion' or eversion. In other women, a ★cervical smear may indicate the presence of abnormal cells, and a piece of tissue will then be taken from the cervix; this shows that the woman has an abnormality, not amounting to cancer, of the cervix. Both conditions may be treated by cauterization of the cervix. This involves burning off the abnormal cells with the tip of a small instrument which has been heated by an electric current. This enables healthy cells to grow over the area when the burned cells have sloughed off. In recent years, cauterization has been replaced by other methods which are more efficient in treating abnormalities of the cervix. One of these, which has become popular, is cryosurgery, in which the surface of the cervix is frozen. The frozen cells die and slough off, causing less discomfort than cauterization. Another method is to 'vapourize' the abnormal cells by means of a laser.

Cellulite

The word 'cellulite' was invented in Europe to make women believe that the fat on their thighs and abdomen is not fat but some other special substance which will disappear if the advertised ointment or recommended massage is used – no valid document supports these claims yet. There is no scientific evidence that cellulite exists: it is simply fat. Unfortunately, fat which is deposited on thighs and abdomen is the last to be burned up when a person diets to lose weight. The treatment of cellulite is the same as treatment of overweight: to diet, to exercise, and – if it makes a woman feel good – to use massage.

Cellulitis, pelvic

In a few cases of pelvic infection, usually following an illegal abortion or at childbirth, the bacteria enter the tissues which surround and support the cervix where they cause an acute infection. If this is not treated it becomes chronic pelvic cellulitis, which causes considerable discomfort. The woman feels a dull ache in her pelvis, intercourse is painful, and examination by a doctor shows that the uterus is also affected. The condition is increasingly rare today, both because legalized abortion is more readily obtainable, and because far greater care is taken at childbirth to ensure infection is avoided, while at the same time potent antibiotics are available to treat acute infection.

Cephalhaematoma

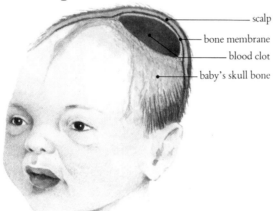

scalp

bone membrane

blood clot

baby's skull bone

A cephalhaemotoma is a blood clot which occasionally forms on the skull of a newborn baby. It is caused either by pressure on the baby's head as it passes through the *birth canal or, more usually, during a *forceps delivery, when the membrane covering one of the bones of the skull is lifted away and a blood clot forms between the membrane and the skull. Although the swelling looks ugly, and stays the same size for 2 or 3 weeks, it slowly dissolves and no treatment is required. As the blood clot is outside the skull, no brain damage occurs.

Cerebral palsy

A number of babies (2 in every 1000 born) who have been severely deprived of oxygen (hypoxic) either in late pregnancy or during childbirth develop signs of a spastic weakness of the legs which may be associated with writhing movements of the hands and arms. The signs may not appear until the child is a year old or later. The lack of oxygen (hypoxia) causes swelling and damage of certain groups of brain cells, which is the reason for the name given to the condition, cerebral palsy. In the past it was thought that cerebral palsy was due to a traumatic childbirth, and this may in fact be the cause in a small number of cases. But in over 90 per cent of 'spastic' children, the cause is severe hypoxia, causing brain damage, in pregnancy or, more often, during labour. Babies which are born *preterm or are of low birth weight are more likely to develop cerebral palsy. With better *fetal monitoring in childbirth, warning signs of severe hypoxia can be detected and corrective action taken, so that the frequency of cerebral palsy should diminish.

Cervical 'erosion'

The *cervix, which projects into the upper part of the vagina, is hollow and its canal joins that of the uterus. The cells which line the canal secrete mucus, especially at the time of *ovulation. The portion of the cervix projecting into the vagina is covered with layers of cells. Under the influence of the hormone *oestrogen, especially at puberty and during pregnancy, the tissues of the cervix swell, and the cells lining the canal are exposed, in a reddened area around the canal. This condition used to be referred to as a 'cervical erosion', but is more correctly called a 'cervical eversion'. It was thought to cause backache, vaginal discharge, and bladder infection, and the treatment was to remove the cells by cauterization. Today, however, it is known that treatment is not needed for a cervical 'erosion' unless the woman has a persistent heavy discharge which is not due to vaginal infection. If treatment is required, then the affected area is either frozen using cryosurgery or it is burned using diathermy. The first method is painless, and is followed by less discharge and better healing than the burning method.

Cervical polyp

The *cervix is the lower part of the uterus and projects into the upper vagina. It is traversed by a canal which is lined with cells arranged as a series of clefts. Occasionally, a part of the tissue between two clefts overgrows, leading to an elongated rounded red mass which pokes out of the cervix. This is a cervical polyp. The woman may develop an increased amount of vaginal discharge or scanty intermittent bleeding from her vagina, which tends to occur after intercourse, but many women have no symptoms. Polyps are usually harmless, but a woman who develops the symptoms described should visit a doctor. If a cervical polyp is found, the treatment is to remove it and examine it under a microscope as a small proportion are cancerous.

Cervical smear

The cervical smear was introduced over thirty years ago by Dr Papanicolaou (hence its other name 'Pap' smear) to detect cancer of the neck (cervix) of the uterus at a stage when it could be completely cured. The smear is taken by exposing the cervix by means of a vaginal *speculum during a *pelvic examination. Some of the cells which cover the cervix are scraped gently from its surface using a wooden spatula or with a cotton-wool swab. These are smeared on to a glass slide, which is immediately placed in a jar of alcohol. This is sent to a laboratory where the slide is stained and examined for abnormal cells. Over 90 per cent of smears show no abnormality; the other 10 per cent are discussed with a pathologist who sends a report to the woman's doctor. This will read 'negative' (meaning the cells are normal); 'atypical' (meaning the smear should be repeated in 6 weeks); or 'positive' (meaning that further investigation of the cervix is needed). This may include examination with a *colposcope and biopsy of the cervix, in which a small amount of tissue is removed from the cervix for examination by a pathologist.

A cervical smear should always be part of a gynaecological examination. Any sexually active woman should arrange to have a smear made. Once she has decided, and had the smear taken, a second smear is taken 6 months later and thereafter a smear need only be taken every 3 years (although it is advisable for women from the age of 40 to have a gynaecological check each year, when a cervical smear could also be taken).

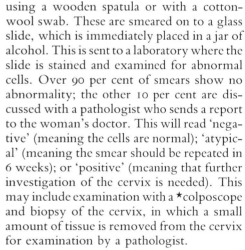

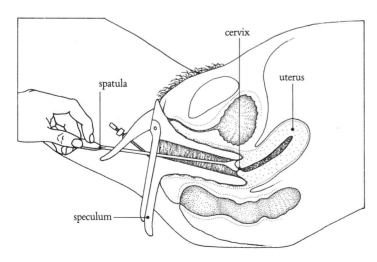

Chancre

A chancre is a hard-edged ulcer which appears on a woman's *vulva (in a quarter of cases on her cervix) if she is infected with *syphilis. The ulcer is round and level, with rolled edges and a soft centre which exudes fluid. It is usually painless. The ulcer develops between 2 and 6 weeks after infection, and lasts for the same period, after which it heals. In most cases the glands in the groin are enlarged. The fluid is alive with spirochaetes, the bacteria which cause syphilis, and in consequence the woman will infect any man with whom she has sexual intercourse during this period.

In tropical countries, another form of chancre, the *soft chancre* (chancroid), may occur. This is caused by infection by a small organism called Ducrey's bacillus. Several ulcers usually occur, 7 to 10 days after intercourse with an infected man. They have soft edges, are very painful, and bleed easily. The

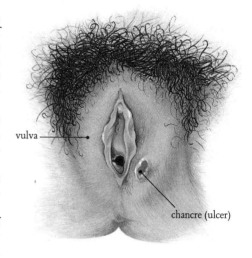

vulva

chancre (ulcer)

glands in the groin are greatly enlarged and matted together to form a big, painful, red swelling. Both types of chancre are treated with antibiotics.

Chastity

In most societies in the past and in many today, women are expected to remain virgins until they marry and following marriage to remain faithful to their husband. If they do not they are punished and the family is shamed. Men, on the other hand, are allowed – often expected – to obtain sexual experience before marriage, and although they are expected to remain faithful after marriage, it is accepted that many have other sexual relationships. In Western society today, the concept of pre-marital chastity is accepted in principle but ignored in practice. Between 50 and 70 per cent of women have sex before marriage. There is no evidence that pre-marital sex is harmful, or that chastity is beneficial to a marriage relationship; and there is no evidence of the reverse. A woman will remain chaste until marriage if that accords with her moral values, her desires, experiences, and learning and if she feels happy in her decision.

Chemotherapy

The development of cytotoxic drugs, powerful medications which kill rapidly dividing body cells, has opened up a new era in the treatment of some forms of cancer: chemotherapy. Cancer cells divide rapidly (as do the cells which line the intestinal tract from the mouth down, and those from which hair develops) and consequently are more vulnerable to these cytotoxic drugs. In the treatment of cancers which affect women exclusively, chemotherapy is given in malignant *trophoblastic disease, in some cases of *breast cancer following surgery, and in cases of *ovarian cancer where the malignancy has spread beyond the ovary. A variety of cytotoxic drugs have been made and they are often given in combination, usually for a few days at a time. Most women feel nauseated or vomit during chemotherapy; some women develop a sore mouth, or diarrhoea, and a few women lose most of their hair. Nausea and vomiting cease when the course of chemotherapy is complete, but may recur with subsequent courses of cytotoxic drugs. When chemotherapy is concluded, the woman's hair regrows.

By using chemotherapy, nearly all women who have malignant trophoblastic disease are cured, and many women who have cancer of the breast or ovary live longer without symptoms. For example, while 45 per cent of women with breast cancer which had spread to the lymph nodes in the armpit were alive and free from cancer 5 years after surgery, the proportion rose to 60 per cent if chemotherapy was given. When chemotherapy is suggested in the treatment of cancer it is usual for the doctor to discuss fully with the patient the type of treatment he proposes, the troublesome toxic side-effects which will probably occur, and how these can be reduced, and the long-term outlook. Most women who have received chemotherapy feel that as the drugs kill cancer cells and improve the chance of survival, they are prepared to accept the side-effects.

Child abuse

Every mother at some time becomes so frustrated and angry with her child that she wants to hit him – and then feels guilty if she does. This is a normal response, but a number of parents treat their children abnormally, hitting them so that their bodies are injured, sometimes severely, or depriving them of love and security so that their minds are abused. These parents are abusing their child. The prevalence of child abuse is unknown, but research studies in Britain and the United States suggest that 6 out of every 1000 babies will have been seriously neglected or physically abused before their third birthday. Many of these babies are physically or mentally handicapped. Many of the mothers show an inability to cope with their newborn baby or to initiate the *bonding process, and often have a history of being abused in childhood. The children more likely to suffer physical abuse are those whose mother was found to be unwilling or unable to care for her newborn baby; who had shown disturbed behaviour in hospital; who had no supportive partner, or relative; or who had severe marital problems. Many of these mothers who are likely to be unable to cope can be identified in the first weeks after childbirth by simple observations by a nurse-midwife. It has been demonstrated that if a supportive, preventive service provided by paediatricians and social workers is made available, then the frequency and severity of child abuse decreases.

Childbirth, estimated date

Every woman who is pregnant wants to know when she may expect the baby to be born. If the woman has regular menstrual cycles, and knows the date on which her last period began, then a quick calculation can establish the date to within 10 days.

The calculation is done by adding 10 days to the date of the first day of her last menstrual period, subtracting 3 months from the month in which it occurred, and adding one year. See the table opposite.

If the woman has irregular or long menstrual cycles, has forgotten the date on which her menstrual period started, or does not see

First day of menstrual period	19 July	1985
Add 10 days	29 July	
Subtract 3 months	29 April	
Add 1 year		1986
Estimated date	29 April	1986

a doctor until after the 15th week of pregnancy, an *ultrasound examination between the 16th and 20th weeks can accurately determine the date her baby will be born.

Childbirth, labour

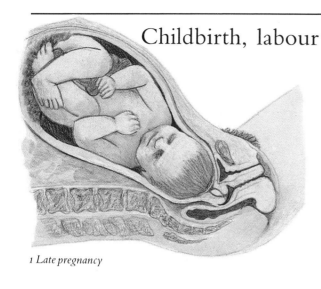

1 Late pregnancy

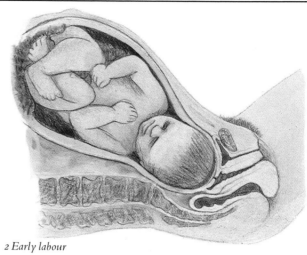

2 Early labour

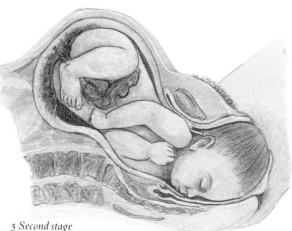

5 Second stage

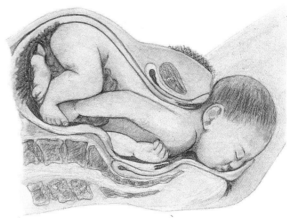

6 Crowning

Traditionally, the process of childbirth, or labour, has been divided into three stages. The *first stage* extends from the onset of labour to the time when the ★cervix is fully dilated, that is its edge is flush with that of the vagina and the rest of the uterus. The *second stage* extends from full dilation of the cervix up to the time the baby has been fully expelled from the mother's body. During this stage the mother's efforts help to push the baby into the world. The *third stage* extends from the birth of the baby until the time the ★placenta is expelled. The table shows the average duration of the stages of labour in hours, and in over 90 per cent of women the duration of labour will fall into this range.

The duration of labour is not necessarily influenced by the age of the woman.

One difficulty with this calculation is that it is not easy to determine the onset of labour with accuracy as the transition from pre-labour (when painful uterine contractions may occur) to labour (when the contractions are regular and occur at decreasing intervals) may be imperceptible. The obstetrician will therefore look for a second indicator: the ★'show', a discharge of bloody mucus from the cervix which appears at the vulva. Occasionally the onset of labour is heralded by a gush of water, as the 'bag of waters', that is the membrane which surrounds the ★amniotic sac and fluid, breaks.

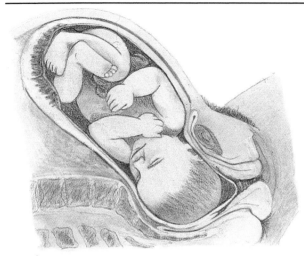

3 Late first stage (membranes intact)

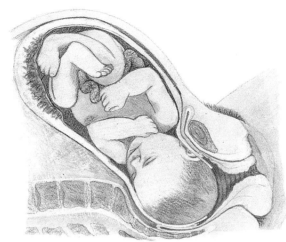

4 Late first stage (membranes ruptured)

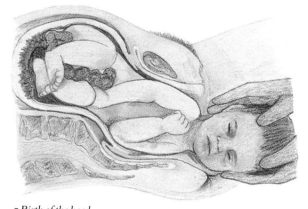

7 Birth of the head

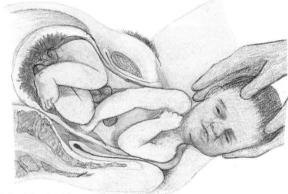

8 Birth of the shoulders

Aware of this inaccuracy, many obstetricians now mark the onset of labour as the time the woman comes into hospital with regular, progressive painful contractions, and a vaginal examination shows that the cervix is dilated by at least 2 cm. It has also been observed that the first stage of labour has two distinct phases. The first, which lasts a variable number of hours, is the *quiet phase* and continues until the cervix is about 3 cm (or three-tenths) dilated. The *active phase* follows normally between 1 and 6 hours, and ends when the cervix is fully dilated (about 10 cm in diameter).

It is currently fashionable to chart the progress of childbirth visually on a chart called a ★partogram.

	First baby		Subsequent baby	
	Average duration	*Range*	*Average duration*	*Range*
First stage	8¼ hrs	(2–12 hrs)	6 hrs	(1–9 hrs)
Second stage	½ hr	(¼–1½ hrs)	¼ hr	(0–¾ hr)
Third stage	¼ hr	(0–1 hr)	¼ hr	(0–½ hr)
	9 hrs	(2¼–12 hrs)	6½ hrs	(1–10¼ hrs)

Childbirth, pain relief

For a few women, childbirth is completely, or almost completely, free of pain. Other women, who have received training by *psychoprophylaxis and are supported during labour by a partner or helper, are able to cope without requiring drugs. However, the majority of women request some form of pain relief in childbirth. In the early part of the active stage of labour, analgesics such as injections of pethidine are usually appropriate; and some very anxious women may also request a tranquillizer. Once the active stage is established and the contractions are strong and painful, the woman has two choices if she wants some form of pain relief. The first is to have one or more further injections of pethidine and to breathe trilene or gas and oxygen with contractions if it is needed later in labour; the second is to have *epidural anaesthesia.

Increasing numbers of women prefer an epidural. A narrow needle is inserted into the epidural space between the two membranes which cover the spinal cord, and an anaesthetic is injected into it. This blocks all (or most) sensations of pain from the uterus, and sometimes the upper parts of the legs. The anaesthetic is added at intervals, as required. Epidural anaesthesia is associated with a higher rate of *forceps deliveries, and a few women may develop a severe headache afterwards.

Women who choose pethidine and trilene may wish to receive further pain relief during the actual birth of the baby. In these cases, a local anaesthetic is injected into the tissues of the *perineum or via the vagina, to block the nerves which supply the area. This is called a pudendal nerve block.

Modern obstetric care stresses the importance of communication between the woman and the health professionals who look after her. A woman needs to know about, and be in a position to choose, in discussion with her doctor or midwife, the form of pain relief she is given.

Child prostitution

In many large cities there are increasing numbers of children aged 9 to 15, of both sexes, who have become prostitutes. In most cases the child has run away from home because of brutal or indifferent parents, and resorts to prostitution to make money, which is spent on cigarettes, drugs, pinball parlours, and movies. In a few cases, however, the child is forced into prostitution by a parent. The most common sexual services offered by boys and girls are masturbation and oral sex. Vaginal or *anal sexual intercourse is less common, although it does occur more frequently if the child is older.

Many of these children have no sense of belonging and experience a feeling of complete rejection. In the city environment they may be exploited by pimps, or may be treated with consideration by a protector. Most of these children become hard but still see their experience as transitory and hope to settle down, although many believe that they will die early and perhaps that relationships are illusory.

Chromosomes

Each body cell contains a jelly-like substance called cytoplasm which surrounds the nucleus. The nucleus of the cell carries all the genetic information needed to create a new individual, in the form of several long 'tapes' of genes which form the chromosomes. The number of chromosomes varies between species; a human cell has 46 chromosomes, which are of various lengths and sizes. Two of the chromosomes determine the sex of the person. There are two forms of sex chromosomes, named X and Y because of their shapes. If a person's body cells contain two X chromosomes (46 XX), the person is female, while if the chromosome complement of the person's body cells is 46 XY, the person is male. It is possible to display chromosomes in a *karyotype enabling chromosomal abnormalities to be detected early. *Down's syndrome is a common chromosomal abnormality in which the chromosome complement of the cells is 47.

Circumcision, female

The *clitoris is the female equivalent of the penis and also has the equivalent of a foreskin. This is the prepuce or clitoral hood. In some Islamic nations, part of the prepuce is removed ritually for religious reasons in childhood, usually between the ages of 5 and 10. In certain countries a much more extensive mutilating procedure takes place. In Egypt, for example, the prepuce, the head of the clitoris, and the adjacent parts of the inner lips (labia minora) are excised. In the Sudan, the most extensive form of female circumcision (Pharaonic circumcision) is practised: the clitoris, the whole of the inner lips, and part of the outer lips are excised, leaving a small opening to the vagina. The operation is carried out by women who have no medical knowledge or training. Severe pain, shock, bleeding, and infection are unavoidable, and a painful scar may persist. The purpose of the ritual procedure seems to be to reduce female sexual desire, so that the woman remains faithful to her husband. In a study made in Egypt of 1000 women who had been circumcised, 30 per cent found sexual intercourse painful or uncomfortable, and had little sexual feeling. Female circumcision is condemned by women's leaders in Islamic nations, but as yet it continues to be performed extensively.

Circumcision, male

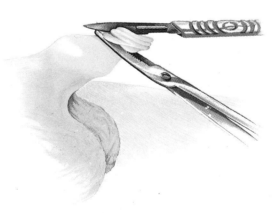

The foreskin protects the penis and there is no valid medical reason for circumcision

Many parents still wonder whether to have their newborn male baby circumcised. All Jewish male babies are circumcised on the 8th day after birth, and Moslem boys are circumcised at puberty. In the 1950s, over 95 per cent of male babies in America were circumcised, most cases because of medical fashion. It was said that 'the mother wanted it, the doctor profited by it, and the baby couldn't complain'. There is no medical reason for circumcision. The reasoning behind the operation, in which the foreskin of the penis is cut off, was that it made the penis cleaner, it prevented the boy masturbating, and it enabled a man to delay ejaculation longer. These reasons have no validity. The foreskin is adherent to the underlying glans, usually until the baby is about 18 months old (in some babies to the age of 5 or 6 years). The penis should be washed under the foreskin after it can be easily drawn back. Circumcision does not prevent masturbation and has no effect at all on a man's sexual performance. There are in fact good reasons for avoiding circumcision: it is known that the operation has been followed by death; and the foreskin protects the penis from becoming inflamed by the ammonia in the baby's urine while he is wearing nappies thus causing unnecessary discomfort.

Cleft palate

Cleft palate and cleft lip (hare lip) occur about once in every 1000 births unless one parent is affected by cleft palate, when the chance increases to about one in 15 births. When the baby is examined at birth, he may be found to have only one condition, or both may occur together. If the cleft is small, feeding may present no problems, but with larger clefts difficulties may arise. It is now normal practice for the baby to be fitted with a plate in the roof of his mouth soon after birth; subsequently new plates are fitted as he grows, and the cleft palate is eventually repaired surgically, usually when the baby is about 15 months old. Hare lip is repaired at an earlier stage when the baby is between 6 and 12 weeks old, and this has excellent cosmetic results.

Clitoral hood, adhesions

The fold of the inner lips (the labia minora) which join together over the *clitoris is called the clitoral hood. The clitoris is the most sensitive erotic zone of a woman's genital organs, and in recent years numerous magazine articles have claimed that adhesions between the clitoral hood and the clitoris reduce sexual feelings and enjoyment. Some physicians have developed operations to 'release' the clitoris from the adhesions – a sort of circumcision.

Recent research has shown that clitoral adhesions are not a cause of reduced sexual feelings. Firstly, they are very rare: in one study only 2 cases of possible adhesions were found in 2000 consecutive examinations. Secondly, there is no evidence that so-called clitoral circumcision increases a woman's sexual response. A very few women have an adherent clitoral hood, and these women suffer pain when the clitoris is stimulated. The adhesions can be freed with surgery.

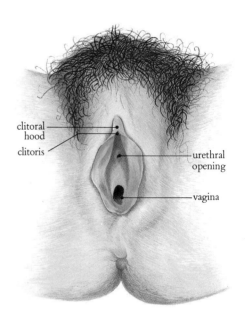

Colostrum

Colostrum is the thick, lemon-yellow liquid which may leak from the nipples in the second half of pregnancy and in the first days after childbirth. It is produced by the milk-secreting cells of the breast, which subsequently secrete mature milk. Compared with mature milk, colostrum contains less fat, less milk-sugar, more protein, and a much higher level of protective antibodies. This suggests that the function of colostrum is to protect the baby from infection. Colostrum may also have a laxative effect. By the fourth day after birth, it is replaced by transitional milk, and then by mature breast milk 5 days later. Abnormal secretions can sometimes occur outside pregnancy.

Colposcope

A colposcope is a portable binocular magnifying device which is used in examinations to exclude ★cervical cancer. The woman lies on her back with her legs apart, and a ★speculum is introduced into her vagina to expose the cervix. The colposcope is placed in front of her vagina and its light directed on to the cervix. The gynaecologist then looks through the binoculars and is able to see the cervix magnified between 5 and 25 times; this enables him to detect abnormalities in the cells which cover the cervix. In expert hands, the colposcope can be used to identify the extent and severity of these changes, and also enables the doctor to obtain samples of tissue from the most suspect areas. These are then sent for examination under a microscope in the laboratory.

Condom

Condoms (also known as French letters, rubbers, and sheaths) are designed to envelop the penis during ★sexual intercourse to prevent unwanted pregnancy. Modern condoms are made of thin latex rubber and are prelubricated. They are individually packaged in sealed aluminium foil sachets, and are available in a variety of colours. The condom is removed from its pack by breaking the foil. Any air is expelled from the end and the condom is unrolled over the entire length of the erect penis shortly before sexual intercourse; this may be done either by the man or by his sexual partner. As the penis shrinks after ejaculation, the man must be careful to avoid any leak of sperms into the vagina, by holding the rim of the condom against the penis when he withdraws. Additional contraceptive protection is provided if the woman inserts a spermicidal foaming tablet or cream (vagitory) in her vagina before intercourse. Condoms are also useful in reducing the spread of some ★sexually transmitted diseases. If a couple use a condom properly and each time they have sexual intercourse only 2 or 3 per 100 women will become pregnant in any year in which this method of contraception is used.

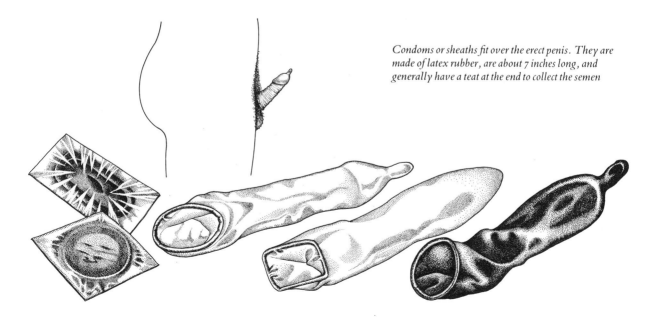

Condoms or sheaths fit over the erect penis. They are made of latex rubber, are about 7 inches long, and generally have a teat at the end to collect the semen

Cone biopsy

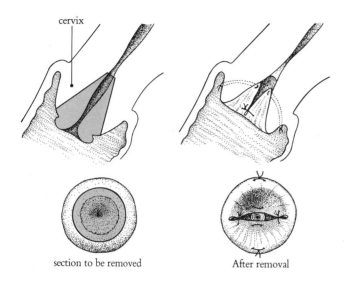

cervix

section to be removed

After removal

The abnormal area of the cervix is excised together with a cone of underlying tissue. The remaining defect is oversewn to reduce bleeding

It is now recommended that ★cervical smears should be made at regular intervals in women between the ages of 20 and 60. The smear is examined in the laboratory and graded as normal, atypical, or suspected of malignancy. If the last type is reported, the test is usually repeated and a second examination made. If this gives the same result, then further action is taken. Many gynaecologists examine the cervix with a ★colposcope, which enables them to identify any areas of abnormal cells. Other gynaecologists carry out a cone biopsy which involves removing the area of tissue containing the abnormal cells by means of a scalpel or a laser beam. The tissue is sliced finely and slices examined under a microscope so that a firm diagnosis can be reached. The operation is carried out under general anaesthesia and the woman has to remain in hospital for between 1 and 5 days afterwards. There is little discomfort, but in about 10 per cent of women bleeding continues after the operation, or recurs in the first 14 days, and this requires treatment. Newer methods have reduced the need for cone biopsy, but it still has an important role in the detection of cervical cancer.

Congenital malformations

About 980 babies in every 1000 are born without any congenital malformation or defect. The remaining 20 have defects of varying degrees of severity. Congenital defects include inherited defects and those caused by infection or problems during the development of the fetus. Chromosomal defects, particularly ★Down's syndrome and ★neural tube defects, together account for half of the total. In some cases, part of the other body systems of the baby may be found to be abnormal, the heart for example. This is usually detected by the doctor who examines the newborn child. In other cases, the gastrointestinal tract may not have formed properly; the baby may have a ★cleft palate or cleft lip; or the oesophagus may not have been formed properly (this is rare, but is usually cured by surgery). Slightly more common is a narrowing of the baby's small intestine just below the stomach, which leads to projectile vomiting. This affects boy babies more than girls and is treated surgically. The baby may be found to have the condition called imperforate anus, where the anus or rectum is closed at the end of the intestinal tract; this also requires surgery. The bones and joints may be affected; the most common disorders are those of the foot (club foot) and congenital dislocation of the hip, which requires splinting. Minor blemishes may be found on the skin; these usually appear in the form of birthmarks.

Nearly all congenital defects are found when the baby is examined soon after birth. If any disorder is identified then the mother and her partner should discuss the most appropriate treatment with their doctor.

Contraception, barrier methods

For centuries women have inserted gums, leaves, fruits, sponges, and similar items into their vagina to block access to the uterus by the sperm and so prevent unwanted pregnancy. Modern barrier methods include the vaginal diaphragm (Dutch cap), the cervical cap and vault cap (Dumas cap); the ★condom is another barrier method, for use by men. In recent years, some women have become disillusioned with the contraceptive ★pill and the ★intrauterine device (IUD), and barrier methods of contraception have grown in popularity.

The *vaginal diaphragm* is the most common method. This is a dome made of latex rubber or plastic mounted on a flexible rim which is reinforced with a metal spring. The diaphragm stretches across the vagina, separating the cervix from the sperm. Because the size of the vagina varies between individual women, the woman has to be examined internally so that she can be fitted with the appropriate size of diaphragm. She will then be taught how to insert the diaphragm and how to withdraw it, and told the correct way to clean and store it. The *cervical cap* and the *vault cap* fit fairly accurately over the cervix and, like the vaginal diaphragm, must also be fitted by a doctor. Some women find them rather more difficult to insert accurately and to remove. The diaphragm is normally used in conjunction with a spermicidal cream or jelly which is smeared on the rim.

The barrier methods of contraception have a number of advantages: their use lies in the woman's control; they can be used during menstruation; they need only be used when needed; they have no significant side-effects; and they may protect against ★cervical cancer. If barrier methods are used properly, the pregnancy rate is low (only slightly higher than with the IUD). The main objection to the barrier methods is an aesthetic one. Some women are not happy about touching their genitals and dislike the idea of inserting an object into their vagina. Another objection is that the man may notice the barrier, or that its insertion interferes with the smooth progress of love-making. This need not be so. The woman may insert the diaphragm in anticipation of making love, or with her partner during ★sexual pleasuring.

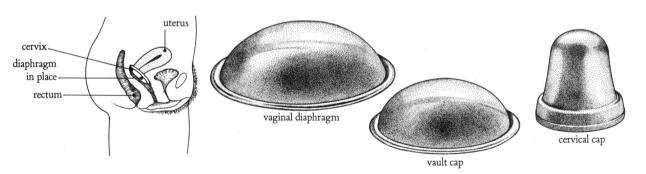

cervix —
diaphragm in place —
rectum —
uterus

vaginal diaphragm

vault cap

cervical cap

Coombs' test

In cases of ★Rhesus iso-immune disease, the red blood cells of the mother absorb rhesus antibodies on certain areas of their surface. This can be demonstrated in a laboratory test, which takes its name from the doctor who devised it. The red cells to be tested are suspended in a solution in a test tube and a substance called antiglobulin is added. If the red cells have absorbed any rhesus antibody, the antiglobulin will adhere to it and the cells will clump together to form granules. A positive Coombs' test indicates that the baby may be affected by ★Rhesus iso-immune disease, and further investigations are required. For instance ★amniocentesis will indicate the degree to which the baby may be affected.

Corpus luteum

Each month during a woman's reproductive years between 10 and 20 *egg follicles grow in the ovary; one of the follicles grows larger than the others and by the 12th to 14th day of a normal menstrual cycle measures between 20 and 25 mm in size. It is from this enlarged follicle that the egg (ovum) will be expelled. Following expulsion of the egg, the follicle collapses and the cells which make up its wall change both in colour, to become yellow, and in function, and produce the hormone *progesterone as well as *oestrogen. It is now called a corpus luteum (yellow body). Unless pregnancy occurs, the life-span of the corpus luteum is short, and only lasts about 16 days. If the egg is fertilized and pregnancy occurs, then the corpus luteum continues to produce hormones for about 40 days.

Cot deaths

Unexplained death of infants has occurred for thousands of years, and the reason why babies die suddenly is still obscure. Cot death – or to give it its official name, Sudden Infant Death Syndrome (SIDS) – occurs more frequently in infants whose parents are young and poor, and if the mother is unmarried. The mother is more likely to be a smoker (or to take hard drugs), to have been ill during pregnancy, or to have lost a baby previously. The baby is likely to have been *premature, *small-for-dates, or a twin.

Cot death occurs most often when the baby is between 1 and 4 months old, in winter, at night, while the baby is asleep in any position. About half of the babies have had a cold or diarrhoea in the week preceding death. About 2 babies in every 1000 born die of SIDS.

A baby suffering from SIDS may die, or may nearly die. If a baby is near death from SIDS it is found asleep, not breathing, blue in colour, and he is unresponsive to gentle stimulation, but starts breathing when vigorously shaken. If he survives the episode, he is at risk of repeating it. There are two ways of dealing with this problem. The first is to keep the baby in hospital under observation for several months. The second is to monitor the baby at home, using an electronic monitor. This has been criticized by some doctors because of the anxiety and stress it creates in some parents. However, most parents who have used monitors at home find that their anxiety is relieved. Monitoring needs to be controlled, however, and the family should be helped by trained medical counsellors.

If the baby dies, the parents need considerable support, as they react with guilt, denial, or hostility, and this places considerable stress on their relationship. Often calm, supportive counselling helps, and recently groups of parents whose babies have died of SIDS have been formed to provide support for others in the same position.

Cramps in legs

The cause of leg cramps is unknown. They can occur at any time of life but are more common in the second half of pregnancy, and tend to occur at night. There is no way of preventing leg cramps but it is said that they occur less frequently if the foot of the bed is raised by 25 cm. Another method which has been used to prevent nocturnal leg cramps is for the woman to take a glass of milk or calcium tablets before retiring to bed. If a cramp occurs during the night it can be relieved by pressing the foot firmly against the footboard of the bed, or preferably, the woman can ask her partner to push upwards on the sole of her foot. Sudden cramp in bed is also a symptom of *varicose veins.

Cravings during pregnancy

Changes in food habits are common in pregnancy. Some women avoid fatty foods, fried foods, or eggs; others go on eating binges and crave sugar-rich foods. A common craving is for fruit; and some women have an urge to eat highly spiced or flavoured foods, such as pickles. Many women hide their food cravings from their partner and satisfy them in secret. The cause of food cravings in pregnancy is unknown, but the craving for spicy foods may be because the woman's sense of taste is dulled. Craving for foods is harmless, but may be expensive. It ceases when the baby is born.

A few women have a craving to eat substances which they would not normally eat. The substances most craved are coal, toothpaste, soap, or clay. If a woman has such a peculiar craving it is called a 'pica' (from the Latin word for magpie).

Cystitis

Cystitis is an infection of the urinary bladder which leads to the need to pass urine frequently and to pain on urination. In most cases, cystitis is caused by bacteria being introduced into the bladder from outside; but sometimes the infection tracks down from the kidney. Cystitis may follow unhygienic toilet habits, particularly wiping the back passage from behind forwards after emptying the bowels. In other cases cystitis follows a flare-up of symptomless bacteriuria. In this condition the bladder is infected by bacteria, but there are no symptoms, until cystitis supervenes. Between 3 and 7 per cent of women have symptomless bacteriuria.

Cystitis may also follow frequent sexual intercourse, particularly if sexual arousal is inadequate and therefore lubrication insufficient. The movement of the penis rubbing the urethra causes bacteria to be transferred up into the bladder. As it used to be believed that women remained virgins until marriage and that during the honeymoon sexual intercourse took place frequently, the condition is sometimes called 'honeymoon cystitis'. A few women continue to have cystitis, long after the honeymoon, each time they have sexual intercourse, the symptoms occurring 12 to 36 hours later. To distinguish it from honeymoon cystitis it is called the 'urethral syndrome'.

The condition can be controlled or cured in two ways. The first is for the woman to drink about 1 litre of water just before intercourse, and to empty the bladder completely 20 minutes later. This has the effect of washing out any bacteria which have been transferred into the bladder. If this does not relieve the condition, a single tablet of nitrofurantoin or trimethoprim taken each evening for several weeks will help.

If a woman has symptoms of acute cystitis which last for more than two days, she should see a doctor. She will be asked to give a specimen of urine, usually collected during 'mid stream' by slipping a sterile container into the flow of urine as she urinates. The specimen of urine is examined in a laboratory and some of it is cultured to determine which bacteria are causing cystitis. The result of the culture enables the doctor to prescribe an antibiotic which will kill the bacteria identified. If no bacteria are grown on culture, the woman does not have cystitis, but is suffering from an *irritable bladder usually caused by psychological problems.

D

Danazol

This drug, which has been recently made available, acts on the pituitary gland, preventing it from releasing the gonadotrophic hormones, that is hormones released by the pituitary gland which stimulate the gonads, or ovaries. Danazol probably also acts directly on the ovaries, preventing the normal release of *oestrogen. Consequently, the woman develops a pseudo-menopause and both ovulation and menstruation cease. The drug has been used successfully to treat *endometriosis and rather less successfully to treat breast pain associated with the *premenstrual syndrome. The main side-effects include acne and oily skin, increased growth of body hair, and swelling of the ankles; about one woman in 10 taking the drug complains of one or more of these side-effects. Once the drug is withdrawn, ovulation and menstruation return within a few weeks.

D and C

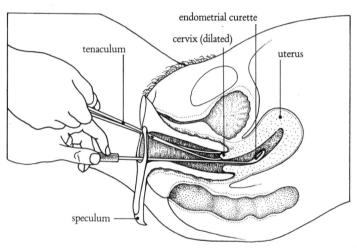

In the surgical operation of curettage, the doctor 'cleans out' the lining of the uterus with an instrument called a curette. A curette is shaped like the rim of a hollow coffee spoon and has a long handle. The *cervix of the uterus has to be dilated (stretched) with graduated metal rods before the curette can be introduced, which is why the operation is called 'dilatation and curettage', or D and C. The lining of the uterus is scraped gently using the curette which brings the tissue through the cervix into the vagina. The tissue is sent to a laboratory for examination.

Curettage is used to remove the remnants of a pregnancy following an abortion, to diagnose the condition of the lining of the uterus (the endometrium) in women who have abnormal menstruation, and, in older women who bleed, to exclude *endometrial cancer.

The operation is carried out under general anaesthetic, and it is usually only necessary for the woman to stay in hospital for half a day. There is no pain after curettage and most women can return to their normal activities the following day.

D and C also means *diagnostic* curettage, which is a better term because it implies that the doctor will send any material curetted from the uterus for examination under a microscope so that a diagnosis is made.

Decidua

The lining of the uterus (endometrium) consists of numerous glands set in layers of cells. If pregnancy occurs, the cells increase in size and the tissues are transformed into a 'decidua' by the actions of the higher levels of *oestrogen and progesterone. The cells of the decidua (the 'soil') are more able to accept the fertilized egg (the 'seed'), which implants in the decidua and grows.

As well as being able to accept a fertilized egg, the decidual cells produce prostaglandins which are involved in the mechanism of *menstruation and of the condition known as *dysmenorrhoea.

Delayed puberty

Puberty is said to have been delayed if by the age of 14 a girl's breasts have failed to develop, or if by the age of 16 she has not menstruated. Most girls who have delayed puberty are shorter and lighter than others of the same age. As part of the investigations of the condition, a careful family history is taken to discover if any other members had delayed puberty. A physical examination is made, including a vaginal examination, and laboratory tests carried out to establish the girl's *karyotype, and to measure certain hormones and bone age. When these investigations have been completed and the results obtained, the doctor will discuss the matter with the girl and her parents, and outline the various types of treatment that are available.

Demand feeding

Mammals – that is animals who breast-feed their young – fall into two categories. Mammals such as deer, dogs, rats, and mice place their young in protected nests or caches, until they are strong enough to fend for themselves. The mother may remain with them, or may wander, returning every 2 to 15 hours to feed the young. Other animals such as cows, sheep, and goats graze constantly and are followed by their young who feed at will, when they feel the need. The composition of the milk produced by the two groups of animals is different. In the first group, the milk is high in protein and often fat; in the second group, the milk is low in both protein and fat. The milk of a human mother resembles that of the second group of grazing animals. This is the reason why most women in primitive societies carry their babies around and allow them to feed on demand.

It is only in recent years that babies have been fed to a schedule and it is now known that the idea was wrong. Babies fed on demand (also called 'need feeding') are less likely to have long crying episodes, thrive better, and are more contented than babies fed to a schedule. After all, the baby knows when he is hungry and wants food.

Dental care

The addiction of many people during childhood to sugar-rich foods and drinks has led to an increase in dental caries (decay) which can only be reversed by good dental hygiene and regular visits to a dentist. The dentist or dental hygienist will be able to give advice on the use of dental floss, plaque-removing tablets, and fluoride tablets, on the correct way to brush the teeth, and on the choice of toothbrush. *Bad breath can sometimes be caused by decay, and a dental check-up will often be beneficial. Pregnancy does not increase the chance of dental caries, and the old belief that 'a child costs a tooth' is untrue. Nevertheless a pregnant woman should visit her dentist early in pregnancy for a check-up.

Deodorants, vaginal

The *vagina is a remarkable organ which is able to clean itself by the action of bacteria which live in it, and its secretions have only a faint odour. If a woman thinks she smells in the vaginal area, it is her pubic hair which is the cause. However, persuasive advertising has induced many women to believe that the smell is due to poor vaginal hygiene and is offensive to other people. Many people are therefore tempted to use a vaginal deodorant. 'Hygienic' vaginal deodorants are neither hygienic nor necessary. They are usually perfumed and may cause irritation in the vagina; in general they should be avoided.

Depression after childbirth

Few people understand that most women find the adjustment to parenthood difficult. Women have been brought up to believe that they should be good housekeepers, excellent lovers, and experienced mothers – all at the same time. Yet when a woman returns home after childbirth, the persistent demands of the newborn baby on her energy, her time, and her emotions can cause considerable stress. The degree and intensity of stress obviously varies, and many women are able to cope with it. In those who are not, the stress is aggravated by modern patterns of family life and the tendency for young people to live at some distance from their close relatives who, in other cultures, were available to offer help and consolation. The stress becomes intensified as the mother realizes that she has the sole responsibility for a small, unpredictable infant who needs attention by day and night. She had not realized that the baby would cry so much, and for so little apparent cause. Her sleep is constantly broken, and fatigue is added to her feelings of inadequacy as a mother. Her relationship with her husband inevitably undergoes a process of adjustment; and this can be emotionally disturbing, particularly if he does not do his share of parenting. As the baby occupies so much of her time, the mother cannot keep the house as clean as she would wish, and feels guilty that she is not the efficient housewife she believed she was.

The fatigue caused by the demands of the baby, the emotional readjustment in her marital relations, the guilt experienced over her untidy house, and the lack of a sympathetic counsellor, can often induce depression. Most women have a short period of emotional upset usually called 'Third-day blues', which occurs during the first week after childbirth, and lasts a few days. One woman in 10 continues to be depressed for a few weeks and in one woman in every 20, the depression becomes so severe that medical help is sought, usually between 2 and 7 weeks after childbirth. The symptoms are mainly changes in moods, predominantly tearfulness, feelings of inadequacy, and inability to cope. These mood changes are unstable, and the depression is usually worse towards evening, when the woman may also complain of fatigue, lack of appetite, and nausea. Certain women are more vulnerable to depression than others: those who were over-anxious or depressed in pregnancy, single mothers or those who have been deserted by their partner, and women who have lost a close relative by death around the time of childbirth.

Doctors frequently offer sedation or antidepressant drugs, when explanation, reassurance, and advice might be far more appropriate. In some cases, antidepressant drugs (particularly tricyclic drugs, such as amitriptyline or doxepin) may be needed; but such drugs should not be prescribed until the doctor has listened to the woman's story and has talked to her about her problems and how she is trying to cope. It is also important that women should know of the community-based organizations which exist; these include the National Childbirth Trust (NCT) and MAMA in Britain, La Leche League International in Britain and the United States, and the Nursing Mothers' Association and Play Groups in Australia. These organizations provide 24-hour home counselling and home visiting when needed. Their activities in helping women to adjust to parenthood can be of great value in reducing the incidence of postnatal depression.

Diabetes in pregnancy

Diabetes complicates about one pregnancy in 400 and a condition of 'glucose intolerance' (gestational diabetes) affects a further 2 per cent of pregnant women (see ★Glucose tolerance test). Pregnancy upsets the treatment of diabetes, as it causes the blood glucose levels to rise and makes control of the condition more difficult.

For this reason a diabetic woman should see a doctor as soon as she thinks she is pregnant so that she may be referred to an obstetrician and a physician with a special knowledge of diabetes. The aims of care in pregnancy are firstly, to maintain the blood sugar in the normal range for as much of the day as possible; secondly, to determine the most appropriate time for the baby to be born; and thirdly, to make sure that the baby is born in a hospital equipped to care for sick newborn babies.

Pregnant diabetic women have to be seen by their doctor at short intervals, and have to keep to a special diet. At each visit, the woman's blood glucose level is measured and the dose of insulin she takes twice daily is adjusted. Women are now being taught to monitor their own blood glucose at home. She may have to spend part of the pregnancy in hospital.

If no complications arise, the pregnancy continues to about the end of the 38th week, when labour may be induced, but action may need to be taken earlier. Special care is taken during labour, which is attended by a paediatrician, who cares for the newborn baby. The baby tends to be overweight and may have problems adjusting to life as he is particularly likely to develop a low blood sugar, and a low blood potassium level. He is also more likely to develop respiratory problems. The baby should be admitted to an Intensive Neonatal Care Unit, where the biochemistry of his blood can be checked regularly, and where the breathing difficulties can be treated effectively. As a result of this improved care and attention, there has been a fall in the number of deaths among babies of diabetic mothers occurring during pregnancy or in the first month of life, and it now stands at between 5 and 10 per cent. As recent as twenty years ago the perinatal loss was as high as 50 per cent.

Diet: a prudent diet

It is clear that the changes in diet that have occurred in the past hundred years have led – at least in part – to what have been called 'diseases of civilization', as they do not usually affect the poorer people in the developing nations. The 'diseases of civilization' include obesity, *high blood pressure, the most common kind of diabetes (non-insulin-dependent, or maturity-onset, diabetes), coronary heart disease, *diverticular disease, appendicitis, *haemorrhoids, hiatus hernia, *varicose veins, *irritable bowel syndrome, and possibly cancer of the bowel and *breast cancer. In the developing countries, only the affluent, who tend to eat a 'Western' type of diet, develop these diseases, and even then, the incidence of the diseases is lower than among people who live in the developed, industrialized countries.

The chances of one or more of these diseases occurring can be reduced if people eat a more sensible diet from childhood onwards. This 'prudent diet' allows people to eat a variety of foods and to have occasional 'feast days' when they can eat anything they like. The principles of the diet are simple and straightforward.

Eat more grains and beans, and more fruit and vegetables, than you have done up to now.

Make sure that the cereal grains used in the food you eat are whole grains; cut down your intake of 'refined' carbohydrates (such as sugar) and of white flour products (bread and cakes).

If you can, eat wholemeal bread. The fibre which it contains assists the activity in your gut, and this in turn prevents constipation and reduces energy absorption from the food you eat. But wholemeal bread is not essential if you dislike it.

Reduce the amount of sugar you eat, and remember that sugar is hidden in many popular foods: cakes, pastries, biscuits, and shortenings.

Reduce the amount of fatty meat you eat; replace it by lean meat, fish, or poultry. Grill or casserole meat and fish, rather than frying. If you do fry fish, do not use any batter – it is mostly made up of carbohydrate.

Reduce the amount of fat you eat, especially the hidden fat in cakes, shortenings, ice-cream, pastries, and biscuits.

You can go on eating butter, but you should spread it thinly.

You can eat eggs, if you enjoy them, but try to keep the number to seven or less a week.

Eat some cheese and drink milk (either on its own, in coffee or tea, or in foods) every day, to provide calcium.

Eat about 120 g or more of green leafy vegetables and some fresh fruit every day.

Reduce the amount of salt in your diet by using table salt very sparingly.

If you eat a sensible, balanced diet and are in good health you probably do not need vitamin or mineral supplements; save your money and buy fresh fruit or vegetables.

Diet in pregnancy

In the years before World War II, the influence of diet on the growth and survival of a fetus was thought to be considerable. Recent studies have now cast doubt on this theory. As far as the obstetrical efficiency of the expectant mother is concerned, the diet she ate in her own infancy and childhood has much more importance. This is the reason why the World Health Organization's Expert Committee on Maternity Care has said that one of the objectives of antenatal care was to help the expectant mother 'learn the art of child care'. This includes teaching her to give her child a properly balanced diet which is rich in protein.

The effect of diet on the outcome of pregnancy has been exaggerated in the past. Fanciful, vague, and complicated diets have been ordered which had little value and were often confusing. In pregnancy a woman has to provide the nutrients which are necessary for the growth of her child, as well as for her own needs. This does not mean that she needs to 'eat for two', and excessive weight gained in pregnancy is very hard to lose after childbirth.

A properly balanced diet provides carbohydrates and fat, which produce the energy needed for life; protein, needed for the formation of new tissues; and vitamins and minerals, which help in the complex chemical processes in the body. All foodstuffs contain one or more of these nutrients. It is unfortunate the cheaper foodstuffs are the energy-supplying carbohydrates, while tissue-building protein, vitamins, and some minerals come from more expensive foods, such as meat. As a result, poorer people, and most people in the developing countries, eat too little protein, vitamins, and minerals,

and barely enough carbohydrate, to cover their daily energy requirements. In the more affluent Western countries, most women eat too much, particularly too much carbohydrate such as bread, cakes, sweets, and sugar, but often eat only just enough protein. Their calorie intake is excessive for their needs, and the excess is stored in the body as fat.

The nutritional needs of a pregnant woman have been considered in great detail by committees in many countries, and the optimal daily allowance for a woman weighing about 55 kg has been worked out. This is set out below.

Calories	2500
Protein	65 g
Calcium	1000 mg
Iron	15 mg
Vitamin A	6000 μ
Vitamin D	400 μ
Vitamin B:	
Thiamine	1.0 mg
Riboflavine	1.5 mg
Nicotinic acid	15.0 mg
Vitamin C (Ascorbic acid)	50.0 mg
Folic acid	0.3 mg

The list can easily be translated into actual foodstuffs, as shown in the table. Briefly, the diet of a pregnant woman should include the following: (**1**) Dairy products: 600 to 900 ml of milk a day, either plain or made up in drinks or used in cooking. Cheese can be substituted for milk if desired (30 g of cheese is equivalent to 250 ml of milk). (**2**) Meat and eggs: 60 to 120 g of lean meat, fish, or poultry a day, and usually an egg. (**3**) Vegetables: green leafy vegetables, which are cooked for less than 10 minutes in a minimum of water, at least three times a week, and other vegetables as desired. (**4**) Bread, cereals, sugar, sweets, potatoes: these provide energy, but when eaten in excess lead to weight gain. Some carbohydrate is needed, but as weight gain has to be monitored during pregnancy, these foods should be eaten in moderation. (**5**) Fruits: an orange or a grapefruit each day, and any additional fresh fruit can be eaten as desired.

Diet, weight-reducing

If you are overweight (see ★Weight, desirable) or are suffering from ★obesity and want to lose weight, you can do this quite efficiently by keeping to a weight-reducing diet and by taking more exercise to increase the amount of energy used. Your chosen diet must be 'balanced', which means that it must provide sufficient quantities of protein, carbohydrate, fat, minerals, and vitamins to keep you healthy. It must also be easy to follow and it must not distort your life-style too much. Energy is needed for bodily functions such as maintaining the body temperature, breathing, digestion, excretion, and to keep the heart beating so that blood circulates round the body. The energy needed for these basic bodily functions varies with body size and composition and amounts to about 6.3 megajoules (1500 kcals) a day. If you want to burn up the energy you have stored in your body as fat, then you should eat a diet producing between 6.3 and 8.4 megajoules (1500 and 2000 kcals) a day. This will permit you to lose about 0.5 kg of weight a week.

A relatively easy diet to follow is one in which all you need do is to count your carbohydrate intake, which should be restricted to between 50 and 100 g a day. An example of this type of diet is set out below.

You can eat as much of the following as you like (but be sensible and recall the principles of a ★prudent diet):

Meat (lean)	Butter
Fish	Cheese
Eggs	Green leafy vegetables

You can eat a limited amount of these foods:

Milk:	up to 600 ml a day
Fresh fruit:	not more than two of the following a day: apples, oranges, grapefruit, pears, peaches; or one of the above and an average serving (about 120 g) of strawberries, raspberries, gooseberries, plums, blackberries, cherries, or grapes

You must restrict these foods because they contain carbohydrate, although you can substitute one for the other:

Bread (preferably wholemeal)	Cornflakes
	Potato, average size
Oatmeal	Baked beans
Biscuits	Nuts

In a day you can have up to three slices of bread (depending on how quickly you want to lose weight) or the equivalent. The number of calories in the following foods is about equal: 1½ slices of bread = 1 average potato = 3 small sweet biscuits = 1 average serving of oatmeal porridge, or cornflakes, or baked beans.

These foods are recommended because they contain the dietary fibre necessary in a diet to keep you healthy.

You must avoid these foods, as they consist either completely or mostly of carbohydrate:

Sugar (raw or refined)

Sweets and chocolates

Jams and honey

Pastries and puddings

Cakes and buns

Canned fruits

Soft drinks (except soda water)

You should avoid alcoholic drinks, but if you cannot, limit yourself to one of the following:

Beer: 250 ml (½ pint)
Whisky: 30 ml (1 measure)
Wine: 125 ml (1 glass)

It may well be that while you are on a diet you are invited out to a dinner party. There is no need to be embarrassed, or to embarrass your hostess, by toying with your food and leaving most of it on the plate. You just have to be sensible and enjoy yourself. Do not eat the bread roll and the pudding unless it is a fresh fruit salad, and limit the amount of alcohol you drink. Only take one potato, but eat everything else. If you *do* exceed your daily quota of carbohydrates, do not let it upset you – return to your diet the next day.

Avoid 'crash' diets and gimmick diets, which appear in women's magazines and as books at frequent intervals. Most of the diets are nutritionally unsound and do not effectively reduce weight (in the short term they may do) or enable you to maintain your weight at the lower level in the long term. Organizations such as Weight Watchers International Inc. and others can be most helpful in providing the motivation to lose weight by dieting and to maintain the new lower weight.

Dildo

A dildo is an object which can be used as a substitute penis for masturbation or for insertion into the vagina. Dildos are usually made of plastic and are available in various shapes including those resembling a penis. Some are hollow so that they can be filled with liquid and squeezed to mimic ejaculation of sperm. A further type of dildo exists, called a *vibrator, which is fitted with an electric vibrating device.

Diuretics

Each day up to 200 litres of fluid are filtered through the kidneys, most being reabsorbed through the kidney tubules beyond the filter (the glomerulus), so that the amount of urine which is actually passed each day is less than 1.5 litres. Diuretics are drugs which reduce the ability of the kidney tubules to reabsorb the fluid, thus larger amounts of urine are passed. Diuretics also reduce blood pressure and they are therefore used to treat people with *high blood pressure, or those who have *oedema, particularly when this is due to heart failure. As a general rule, they should be avoided during pregnancy as the slight swelling of the ankles which many women experience is quite normal. For some years diuretics were used to prevent, and also to treat, *pre-eclampsia, but this has ceased as the drugs did not have any effect on the disease and were detrimental to the fetus.

Diverticular disease

Diverticular disease, which is also called diverticulosis (or, when infection occurs, diverticulitis), most commonly affects the large intestine, especially the lower part of the colon. The disease seems to be increasing in frequency in developed Western countries, especially among older people. This may be due to the fact that they have eaten a diet lacking in fibre for a number of years. The lack of dietary fibre is thought to be

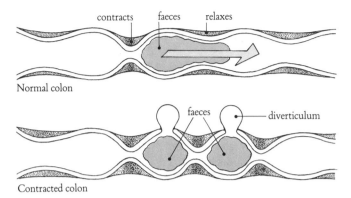

Normal colon

Contracted colon

In the top illustration pressure builds up in one segment of the bowel, one side remains contracted while the other relaxes allowing the contents to be pumped into the next segment. While in the illustration below both sides of the segment contract slowing down the movement of faeces which leads to higher pressure on the wall and bulging

responsible for an increase in the pressure within the gut, and this leads to bulging of weaker parts, which form small pouches, rather in the way small pouches bulge out of an old rubber inner-tube. The person may complain of flatulence, dyspepsia, and persistent pain or discomfort in the lower left part of the abdomen which may be associated with alternating bouts of constipation and diarrhoea, or increasing constipation. The diagnosis is guessed from the person's history and confirmed by X-rays. Treatment is to alter the diet to provide plenty of fibre in the form of wholemeal bread, porridge, fruit, vegetables, and additional bran (if desired). The amount of bran taken should start at 2 teaspoonsful (or two 2 g tablets) three times a day. After 2 weeks, the daily amount should be gradually increased until the bowels can be opened twice a day without straining. In the first weeks of taking bran the person may complain of flatulence but this ceases after a while. Sometimes 'bulk producers' may be prescribed to increase the volume of the motions, which in turn reduces the pressure within the bowel.

Douching

Vaginal douching has never been fashionable outside the United States, and its popularity there is diminishing. The idea behind it was that if the vagina was washed out using a perfumed mild antiseptic solution or a home-made douche of warm water and vinegar, then the woman would feel and be clean. This idea was based on a false premiss. The vagina is self-cleaning because its cells make a dilute acid which controls bacterial growth. It is true that the secretions of the vagina have a faint fishy smell, but this is not noticeable to other people. A second reason for douching was in order to 'clean' the vagina after sexual intercourse, but this is also unfounded as sperm are sterile, and most women make sure that the man's penis is clean before sex.

If a woman feels more comfortable by douching at periodic intervals, using a mild antiseptic, water and vinegar, or water and baking soda, then it probably does no harm, but it does nothing to improve her health.

Down's syndrome

Children born with Down's syndrome (mongolism) are intellectually handicapped, although the degree of handicap varies. They used to be called 'mongols' because their eyes slant, and their head is short on a thick neck. The condition is due to chromosomal abnormality, the baby's cells containing 47 chromosomes instead of the usual 46. The chance of a couple having an affected baby increases from less than one in 1000 if the woman is under the age of 30 to over one in 50 if she is over 40.

The condition can be diagnosed in early pregnancy, and screening by *amniocentesis is offered to all women aged 35 and over. A sample of amniotic fluid is obtained at the 15th week of pregnancy, by introducing a hollow needle into the uterus. Cells from the fluid are grown in a laboratory, and 14 to 21 days after taking the sample, a report is given

Down's syndrome
Drugs in pregnancy
Dysmenorrhoea

which tells whether the fetus is affected with Down's syndrome. If the fetus is affected, the couple can then decide after counselling whether or not they wish the woman to have an abortion, and so avoid the birth of an intellectually handicapped baby.

Drugs in pregnancy

As a general principle, a pregnant woman should avoid all medications unless they are really required. Most drugs will not harm the fetus, although small quantities of the drug do pass through the placenta. A few drugs can cause problems in the fetus in the uterus.

Type of drug	Name	Effects on fetus
Antibacterials	Tetracycline	Yellowing of first crop of teeth
Anticoagulants	Dicoumarin	Increase in fetal defects
	Warfarin	Possible bleeding
Anticonvulsants *(in late pregnancy)*		Possible haemorrhage in unborn baby
Antithyroid drugs		May cause fetal goitre
Benzodiazepines	Valium Librium	Given in large doses in labour may cause the baby to have poor muscle tone for a few days

Dysmenorrhoea

Dysmenorrhoea (painful periods) affects between 15 and 25 per cent of women, with a peak incidence between the ages of 15 and 25, when over 50 per cent complain of period pains, which are severe in 15 per cent of cases. Dysmenorrhoea may incapacitate the woman for two or more days a month, or in milder cases merely make life uncomfortable. The cramp-like uterine pains are felt in the pit of the stomach, but pain may radiate into the back or down the inner side of the thighs. In severe cases vomiting and/or diarrhoea may occur.

The cause of dysmenorrhoea has recently become clearer. It usually occurs only in menstrual cycles during which *ovulation has taken place; anovulatory menstrual cycles, when ovulation has not occurred, are usually painless. The uterine pain is due to spasms of the uterine muscle; this is caused by the hormone *prostaglandin (PG) which is secreted by the lining of the uterus. The quantity of prostaglandin which is secreted varies, as does the sensitivity of the uterine muscle to the hormone. For this reason some women do not experience dysmenorrhoea, some have severe dysmenorrhoea, and others find that the severity of the pain varies from month to month.

Treatment is either to use drugs which suppress the synthesis of prostaglandin; or to prevent ovulation. If the first form of treatment is chosen, then aspirin helps when the period pains are mild, but when the pain is more severe, specific anti-prostaglandin drugs (such as naproxen, or one of the fenamic acids) provide considerable relief. The alternative is to prevent ovulation by means of the contraceptive *pill. The anti-prostaglandin drugs are taken from the onset of the pain for 3 to 5 days, while the pill has to be taken for 21 days every month.

E

Eating disorders

Eating disorders include ★anorexia nervosa, ★bulimia (binge-eating), and gross ★obesity. While obese people are easily identifiable, anorexia nervosa is only obvious in its later stages, and binge-eaters are often not detected. Treatment is more effective if the eating disorder is detected early, particularly if the person has anorexia nervosa or is a binge-eater. Unfortunately, problems may arise as not enough is known about 'normal' eating behaviour, and in consequence, women referred to a doctor may be subjected to either too much or too little investigation, or they may be converted into being a 'patient' who learns to behave in accordance with her 'illness'.

Eating habits in pregnancy

Pregnancy changes the eating habits of many women. In the first 10 weeks, many women are nauseated or vomit, and their appetite is reduced. After this time most women report an increased appetite and are more thirsty. Many pregnant women avoid certain foods (such as fried or fatty food) which they previously enjoyed; other women desire salty foods. Some women find that they can no longer drink coffee or tea. In contrast, many pregnant women have particular ★cravings to eat highly flavoured or savoury foods, fruit, or vegetables, and a few find they want to eat non-food substances.

Provided a pregnant woman eats a mixed ★diet, spending more on fresh fruit, vegetables, and meat, and less on cakes and sweets, she can eat what she chooses. Strict diets should only be chosen for strong medical reasons. Most pregnant women continue to eat the same sort of foods they ate before they became pregnant, but avoiding those foods for which they have now developed a particular aversion.

Eclampsia

The term 'eclampsia' (from the Greek word meaning 'like a lightning flash') was introduced into obstetrics to describe the sudden onset of fits and unconsciousness in a woman in late pregnancy. Eclampsia is almost always preceded by a period when a pregnant woman's blood pressure rises, when protein appears in her urine, and when her body swells (★pre-eclampsia). Eclampsia now occurs rarely in the Western developed countries because of the general acceptance of good ★antenatal care, but it is still common in the developing nations where it is a major cause of maternal death.

Ectopic pregnancy

Ectopic (or tubal) pregnancy occurs when the fertilized egg implants outside the uterus, usually in one of the Fallopian tubes (oviducts), but very rarely on the ovary, or even more rarely in the abdominal cavity. Ectopic pregnancy occurs about once in every 200 pregnancies, but the condition is more common if a woman has previously experienced an infection of her Fallopian tubes, or if she has had surgery to reverse a sterilization operation.

The first indication is that the woman usually has some lower abdominal pain which may become severe. In most cases she has missed a menstrual period, but in 20 per cent of women this may not be so. Following the episode of pain, a small amount of brownish vaginal bleeding occurs. In some cases the woman collapses in shock as a result of a considerable loss of blood inside her abdomen as the ectopic pregnancy erodes a blood vessel.

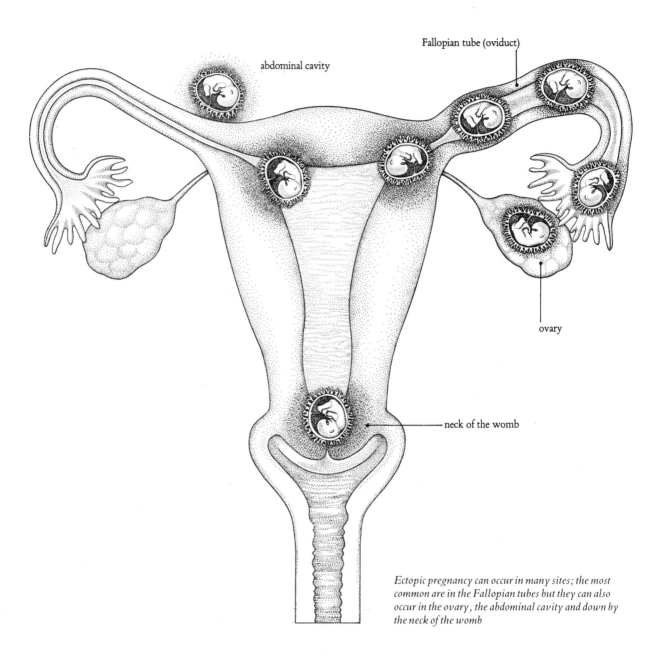

abdominal cavity

Fallopian tube (oviduct)

ovary

neck of the womb

Ectopic pregnancy can occur in many sites; the most common are in the Fallopian tubes but they can also occur in the ovary, the abdominal cavity and down by the neck of the womb

The diagnosis is confirmed by the doctor, either by making an ★ultrasound picture, or by looking inside the abdominal cavity with a ★laparoscope. Another method is to insert a needle into the space between the rectum and the upper vagina; if blood is found, the diagnosis of ectopic pregnancy is likely. Treatment is surgical: usually the ruptured tube containing the ectopic pregnancy is removed, although it can be saved.

Egg follicle

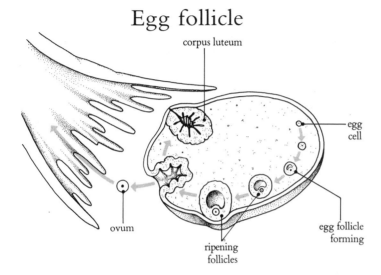

corpus luteum

egg cell

ovum

ripening follicles

egg follicle forming

From about the age of 16 to the age of 45 and less frequently in the years between puberty and 16 and 46 and menopause, each month between 11 and 20 of the egg cells in the ★ovaries start growing. One of them (occasionally more) grows more rapidly, and fluid appears inside the cell separating the egg from the wall of the cell, except at one place. The egg cell has now become a little sac (containing an egg or ovum). The little sac is called a follicle.

This diagram shows the progression of the growing follicle from early in the menstrual cycle until day 14 when the follicle ruptures to release the ovum

Embryo

This is the name given to the new individual from 3 days after fertilization until all the major structures and organs in its body have been formed. This usually occurs by the 50th day after fertilization, or by the 9th week after the last menstrual period. After this it is called a ★fetus.

In the first 3 days the fertilized egg divides recurrently, first to form a ball of cells which look like a mulberry; this is called a morula. A cavity appears in the ball of cells, and fills with fluid. This splits the mass into a 'shell' of cells, with an inner mass of cells several layers thick which cover about one-third of the shell and project into the cavity. The egg is now called a blastocyst. The embryo develops from the inner cell mass, and the ★placenta from the 'shell'.

The development of the embryo is very rapid, and it passes through a stage when it looks like a reptile (4½ weeks), to one when it looks like a monster (6½ weeks), to one when it is recognizably human (8½ weeks). See illustration (at 9 weeks) on page 76.

Endometrial biopsy

Occasionally in the course of investigations for infertility, or during hormonal treatment of menopausal symptoms, the doctor may wish to examine a sample of the lining of the uterus (the endometrium) under a microscope. Using a narrow instrument it is possible to take the sample with relatively little pain, without the need to admit the woman to hospital or to give an anaesthetic. The woman lies on her back, with her legs apart, and the doctor introduces a vaginal ★speculum into her vagina. This exposes her cervix. He then steadies the cervix and slips the instrument into the cavity of the uterus. He withdraws the instrument, taking a tiny strip of the endometrium with it.

75

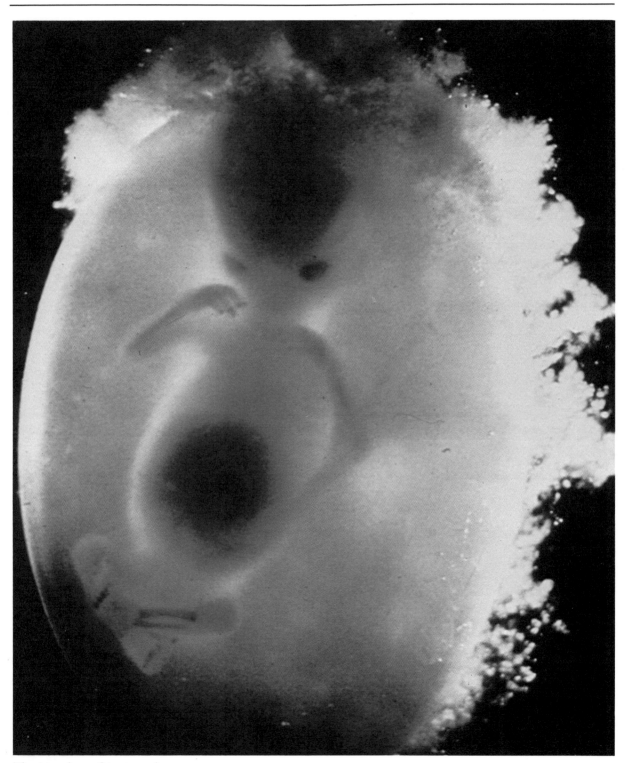

The picture shows a fetus at 9 weeks

Endometriosis

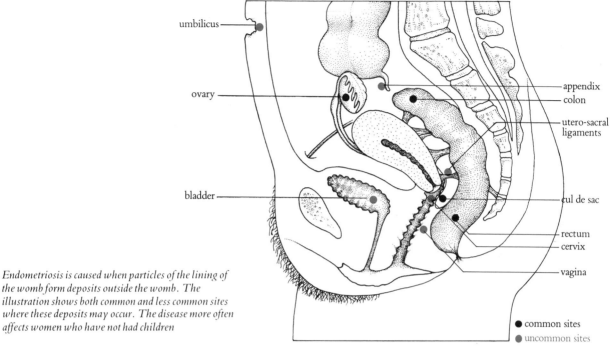

umbilicus

ovary

bladder

appendix
colon
utero-sacral
ligaments

cul de sac

rectum
cervix

vagina

● common sites
● uncommon sites

Endometriosis is caused when particles of the lining of the womb form deposits outside the womb. The illustration shows both common and less common sites where these deposits may occur. The disease more often affects women who have not had children

This disease is caused by the growth of tiny pieces of the lining of the uterus (the endometrium) either deep in the uterine muscle or in other parts of the pelvis. If the tissue grows into the muscle of the uterus, the disease is sometimes called adenomyosis. If the fragments of endometrium reach the pelvic cavity by migrating along the Fallopian tubes (oviducts), the disease is called endometriosis. Often fragments of endometrium grow on the ovary or the outside of the Fallopian tubes, and less commonly in other places in the pelvis. The fragments of endometrium form tiny cysts, and each behaves like a miniature uterus, with bleeding occurring into the cyst when the woman menstruates. As the blood cannot escape (although the serum is absorbed), the cyst slowly increases in size, and is filled with tarry blood. The cysts range in size from a pinhead to a grapefruit. Many women have endometriosis without being aware of it as they do not have any symptoms, except that they are occasionally infertile. Some women develop irregular menstruation or painful menstrual periods, the pain increasing as menstruation continues, to reach a peak on its last day. Other women complain of pain deep in the pelvis during sexual intercourse.

The severity of the symptoms bears no relationship to the extent of the disease. Small areas of endometriosis can be very painful, and large cysts may be painless. A doctor may be able to diagnose endometriosis from the woman's history and by examination, but often he will carry out a laparoscopy. The ★laparoscope enables him to look at the pelvic organs directly and to determine the extent of the disease. In moderate cases, hormone treatment is often successful in curing the disease, but more severe cases require surgery as well. The most successful of the hormones used to treat endometriosis is ★danazol. It has to be taken by mouth each day for between 3 and 12 months, depending on the response. Symptoms are usually relieved in 2 to 6 weeks, and the areas of endometriosis disappear in 3 to 6 months. During treatment most women find that menstruation ceases, their skin becomes more oily, or acne appears, and a few women gain weight.

Epidural anaesthesia

Epidural anaesthesia is a method of relieving pain in childbirth. The nerves which carry pain sensations from the uterus reach the lower part of the spinal cord, while the nerves carrying the impulses which cause uterine contractions leave the spinal cord higher up. If a doctor injects a controlled amount of anaesthetic into the space between the two membranes which cover the spinal cord, pain sensation will be blocked without much effect on the woman's movements. However, she will feel some numbness in her thighs. In this way childbirth becomes painless. The injection is not usually made until labour is fully established (in the 'active' phase; see ★Childbirth, stages of labour), and may need to be repeated before the baby is born. A needle is pushed into the space between the two covering membranes of the spinal cord (the epidural space) in the lower part of the back and a thin plastic tube is threaded through the needle, which is then removed. The anaesthetic is injected through the tube as required.

Epidural anaesthesia is becoming increasingly popular in childbirth, and in many hospitals over half the women choose to have an epidural. A few women develop a headache afterwards, and a ★forceps delivery may be necessary because the woman is less able to push the baby out.

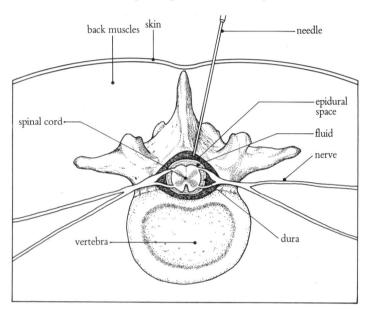

back muscles · skin · needle · epidural space · fluid · nerve · spinal cord · vertebra · dura

During an epidural the anaesthetist inserts a thin needle through the tissues of the mother's back and places the tip in the epidural space between the dura and the bone

Episiotomy

An episiotomy is a cut which is made in the perineum of a woman just before the baby is born when the head is stretching the tissues at the bottom of the vagina. The episiotomy is made to avoid the surrounding tissues tearing. It is normal practice for the doctor to inject a local anaesthetic either before making the incision or after the birth of the baby before stitching the cut.

Following the birth of the baby and the expulsion of the placenta, the episiotomy is stitched. There are several ways of stitching an episiotomy, but all are followed by some discomfort which usually only lasts for 2 or 3 days. The degree of discomfort is dependent to some extent on the size of the episiotomy, the skill of the surgeon, and the type of stitching used.

In 1980 the National Childbirth Trust published two reports on episiotomy from questionnaires sent to 1800 women. They found that an episiotomy had been made in between 60 and 70 per cent of women, and in some cases it was their opinion that the operation had been done for dubious reasons. Over half the women considered that the cut was made before the natural forces of childbirth had adequately stretched the perineum and it was still thick. A second complaint was that many obstetricians did not tell the woman they were about to make an episiotomy and were insensitive to the discomfort it caused during the healing process. In fact many women complained that the pain involved in making the episiotomy, in stitching it, and during its healing period was

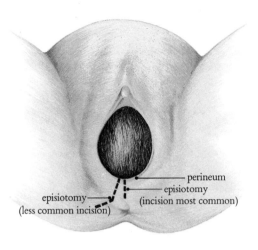

An episiotomy – an incision is sometimes made to help the baby's head to be born safely and to prevent tearing the mother's tissues

severe. It made sitting uncomfortable for days, and the early resumption of sexual intercourse impossible or painful for weeks. In the study one woman in every 5 complained that painful intercourse persisted for more than 12 weeks, and in some it was still present at the time of the survey.

Episiotomy is a beneficial operation if performed appropriately, that is when a stretched perineum is in danger of tearing, or if the baby needs to be delivered urgently by forceps. The NCT reports suggest that a woman should discuss episiotomy with her obstetrician during pregnancy, so that she knows his attitude to the operation, to make sure he will tell her before he makes the episiotomy, and discuss with her what effects she may expect when he has stitched the incision.

Extramarital sex

In most societies, extramarital sex (or adultery) is condemned, and sometimes the participants are punished by the State. This is the situation in fundamentalist Islamic nations. In Western Europe, extramarital sex is not approved of but is condoned, particularly when the husband forms a relationship, and is discreet about it. Extramarital relationships by wives are less acceptable. Most extramarital relationships are discreet and, the extent of the practice is therefore unknown, but it is estimated that at least 40 per cent of married men (and an unknown number of women) have had at least one extramarital affair.

A few couples agree that either or both partners may have extramarital affairs and claim that if they abide by the 'rules' which confirm that their marriage is the primary sustainable relationship, then the affairs are beneficial and increase their love and affection for each other. In most instances, however, an extramarital affair is destructive to the relationship, and one or other of the marriage partners suffers. The wife may suffer pain because of being deceived, cheated, and fooled. She may feel pain because she is rejected and does not know the reason. Her pride is hurt, particularly if her husband's relationship is open, and she may feel that her husband's lover has stolen him from her. Her husband may also be under stress, both emotionally and financially. If the wife begins an extramarital affair which is eventually known to the husband, his masculine pride may be hurt considerably, causing him to question his worth as a man, and a lover.

It should be said that if the marriage relationship is strong and the partners are able to communicate easily and comfortably, any problem which arises between them can be solved, and recourse to an extramarital affair is unlikely. If the relationship is not particularly stable, and moral and religious prohibitions to adultery are not observed, then one of the partners may enter an extramarital relationship. In a few cases, an extramarital relationship is fulfilling and rewarding, but more often than not it will lead to much bitterness, remorse, and jealousy, and many such affairs end in disillusionment and disappointment.

Face presentation

About once in every 500 births, when labour begins the baby's head is not in the usual position, and he lies with his face coming first, rather than the back of the head. In most cases, labour proceeds normally, and the baby emerges from the vagina face first. In about 10 per cent of cases, however, complications occur which mean that the baby has to be delivered by *forceps or *Caesarean section. The baby's face becomes swollen and bruised during labour, and although this may distress the mother when she first sees her baby, the discoloration and swelling disappear completely within a few days.

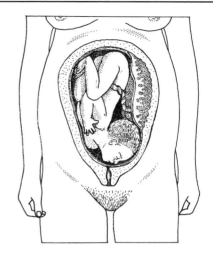

False labour

In the last weeks of pregnancy, the uterus becomes increasingly sensitive and many women complain of painful uterine contractions. These occur at irregular intervals and are more common at night. Although the uterus contracts, the cervix fails to dilate, and for this reason the condition is called 'false labour'. In contrast to true labour, the uterine contractions do not become increasingly frequent and more intense.

False pregnancy

In this bizarre condition (medically known as pseudocyesis) the woman's menstruation ceases, her breasts enlarge and become heavy, and often cloudy fluid can be expelled from the nipples. The abdomen enlarges and the woman is convinced that she is pregnant. However, the pregnancy test is negative and an *ultrasound picture shows a non-pregnant uterus. False pregnancy is a psychological problem, and demonstrates the effect of the mind on the body. The woman needs help and sympathetic advice from a trained counsellor or therapist when the diagnosis has been made.

Fern test

A fern test determines whether *ovulation has occurred. A sample of mucus taken from the *cervix in the middle of the menstrual cycle is smeared on to a dry glass slide. When the mucus dries it may form a fern pattern. If ovulation has occurred, this disappears. Its persistence in samples taken in the second half of the cycle suggests a woman is not ovulating. The test has been superseded in most clinics and instead the blood level of *progesterone is measured on day 20 of the cycle; a raised level indicates ovulation.

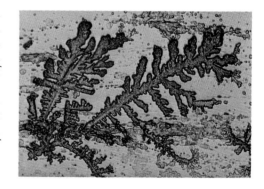

Fertile period

This is the period around the time of ★ovulation when a woman is most fertile. It has been calculated that if a woman has intercourse during the fertile period, she has a 60 per cent chance of becoming pregnant in any one cycle. The fertile period can be detected by checking the secretions of cervical mucus just inside her vaginal entrance each day. When the secretions are clear, slippery, and stretch easily between the fingers, then the woman is in her fertile period. The peak of the fertile period is ovulation, which can be detected in several ways. See ★Natural family planning: the mucus method.

Fertility control

The development in the past fifty years of safe, effective contraceptives, and the increased availability of safe, legal ★abortion, has meant that for the first time in history, a woman can control her fertility and, in consultation with her partner, can decide how many children she wants and when she wants to have them. Fertility control is a matter of choice; the woman and her partner choose which method of ★contraception is most appropriate for their needs, and are confident that, should the method chosen fail to prevent pregnancy, she can obtain an abortion without losing her dignity and will know that it will be performed by a skilled person in a well-equipped, hygienic environment. This has resulted in a considerable reduction in the numbers of women suffering from the results of illegal, infected abortions, a situation which continues to occur in many countries where contraceptives and safe abortions are not easily available.

The effectiveness of the various methods of fertility control can be expressed as the number of pregnancies occurring per hundred women per year (HWY). The smaller the figure, the more effective the chosen method. The table below gives some representative figures for the different methods of contraception.

Method of contraception	Pregnancies per HWY	Method of contraception	Pregnancies per HWY
Most effective		*Highly effective*	
Tubal ligation; vasectomy	0.01 (1 in 10000)	IUD	2.0
Combined oral contraceptives (the pill)	0.05 (1 in 2000)	Injectable gestagens/ Mini-pill	2.0
Sequential oral contraceptives	0.25 (1 in 400)	Diaphragm or condom All users	5.0
		Motivated users	2.0
		Natural family planning All users	20.0
		Highly motivated users	5.0
Less effective		*Least effective*	
Withdrawal	30.0	Post-coital douching	45.0
Vaginal foam or cream	30.0	Prolonged breast-feeding	45.0

Method of fertility control	Deaths per 1 000 000 women	
	Age 25	Age 35
None (i.e. all deaths due to pregnancy)	65	150
Legal abortion (less than 12 weeks)	15	20
The contraceptive pill: non-smokers	15	30
smokers	16	120
IUD	10	15
Diaphragm or condom with legal abortion for failure	15	35
	2	2

The safety of fertility control methods can be calculated from the estimated number of deaths of women each year associated with fertility control per 1 000 000 fertile women. The calculation includes deaths associated with pregnancy if no contraceptive is used or if the method fails. Two examples are given: one for women aged about 25 and the other for women aged 35 (all figures are rounded to the nearest whole number).

Many people may be surprised that the safest method of fertility control is the use of a diaphragm or a condom, with the 'back-up' of legal abortion performed in the first 12 weeks of pregnancy.

Fetal death

By International agreement by the World Health Organization the death of a baby of 500 g or more in the uterus during pregnancy or childbirth is recorded as a fetal death.

In Britain and other developed countries, between 8 and 12 babies in every 1000 reaching the end of the 20th week of pregnancy (when the baby weighs 500 g) will die in the uterus, three-quarters dying before the onset of labour. Most of these babies are of low birth weight (less than 2500 g) and are born prematurely (before the 37th week), often very prematurely. Over half of the, babies have congenital abnormalities, and would not have survived if born alive. Between 1 and 3 babies in every 1000 die during childbirth.

The distress to the parents when their baby is born dead is considerable, and doctors now realize the importance of helping them to cope with their grief and of explaining the reason for the death, in order to dispel any feelings of guilt. Luckily, most couples whose baby is stillborn will have a normal, healthy liveborn baby in any subsequent pregnancy.

Fetal distress

During labour, the doctor or nurse who is attending the birth listens to the baby's heartbeat at regular intervals. If the heart beats too fast or too slowly, or if the amniotic fluid is found to be green in colour when the *waters break, the baby is said to have 'fetal distress', and action is taken to deliver it. However, these clinical signs of fetal distress are not very accurate, and if they are found, it is now usual practice for doctors to use a *fetal heart monitor in order to confirm or deny the diagnosis.

Fetal growth

A baby starts as a single fertilized cell the size of a pinpoint, and grows over a period of about 266 days to become a developed, living organism composed of several billion cells arranged into organs, muscles, tissues, and enclosed in skin, which is 8 million times

Fetal growth
Fetal head, engagement
Fetal head, positions in labour
Fetal heart monitor

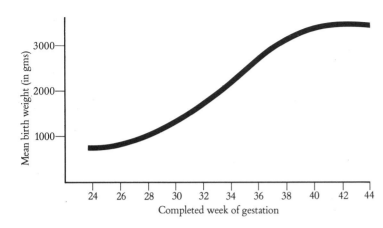

heavier in weight than the original fertilized egg at the beginning of the pregnancy.

In the first 50 days after fertilization (9 weeks after the last menstrual period), when most of the developmental changes occur, the baby is called an ★embryo; after the 50th day it is called a ★fetus. The growth of the fetus can be charted by ★ultrasound, or more usually and less expensively by feeling the mother's abdomen to see how much it is growing. If the growth rate falters, so that the baby becomes ★'small-for-dates', investigations are carried out and a ★fetal heart monitor is used to assess the well-being of the fetus.

Fetal head, engagement

'Engagement of the fetal head' means that at some time in the last 3 or 4 weeks of pregnancy, the baby's head usually settles to lie inside the mother's pelvic bones. Engagement of the head means that its widest diameter (that is, of the skull just above and behind the ears) has passed through the circle of pelvic bones which mark the inlet to the pelvis.

In women carrying their first baby (primigravidae) the fetal head usually engages in the pelvis between 2 and 4 weeks before childbirth. In women who have given birth before (multigravidae) engagement of the fetal head may not occur until a week before childbirth, or until labour begins.

When a doctor examines the woman's abdomen he finds the head is now 'fixed' in the pelvis and relatively immobile. A vaginal examination will show the fetal head occupies much of the inside of the pelvis.

Fetal head, positions in labour

For descriptive purposes, each area of a baby's head is given a special name. For example, the area at the back of the head is called the occiput, and this is usually the lowest part of the baby's head in labour, because the baby keeps its head flexed on its chest. During labour the mother may hear a nurse saying that the baby is a left or right occipito-transverse – she will say it is a 'LOT' or 'ROT'. This indicates the position of the occiput in relation to the bones of the pelvis, viewed from above. The fetal head changes positions as it descends through the pelvis until in 95 per cent of cases the head will be in an OA (occiput anterior) position for delivery. See diagram overleaf.

Fetal heart monitor

Electronic machines have been developed which enable the obstetrician to evaluate the well-being of the fetus in pregnancy and in labour, by observing the pattern of its heartbeats. The machine picks up the heartbeats by means of a device placed on the woman's abdomen or, during labour, by an electrode placed on the baby's scalp after the ★waters have broken. The heartbeats are electronically printed on to a paper moving at a slow speed on the monitor, and show patterns which indicate to the doctor that the baby is not in any danger, or that it may be wise to deliver it quickly.

In pregnancy, the procedure is called ★cardiotocography. Women whose babies are

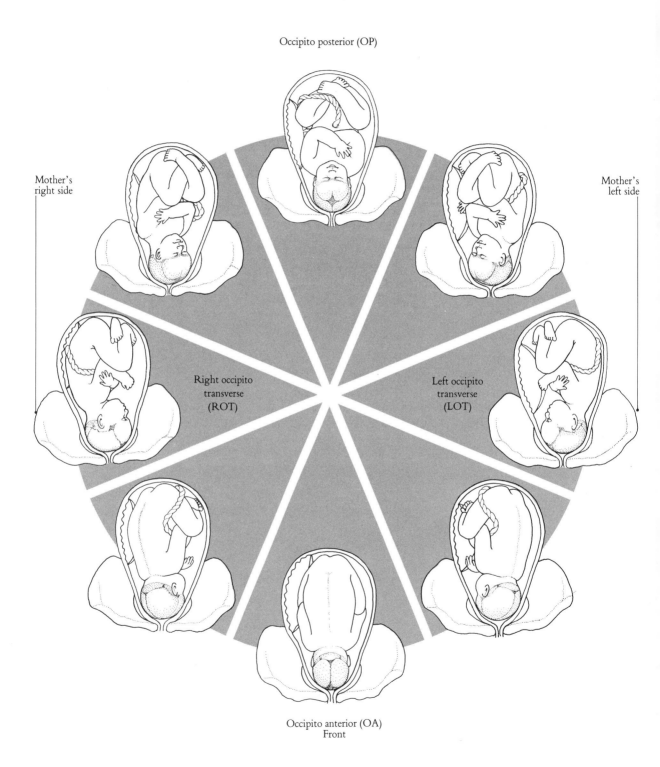

Occipito posterior (OP)

Mother's right side

Mother's left side

Right occipito transverse (ROT)

Left occipito transverse (LOT)

Occipito anterior (OA)
Front

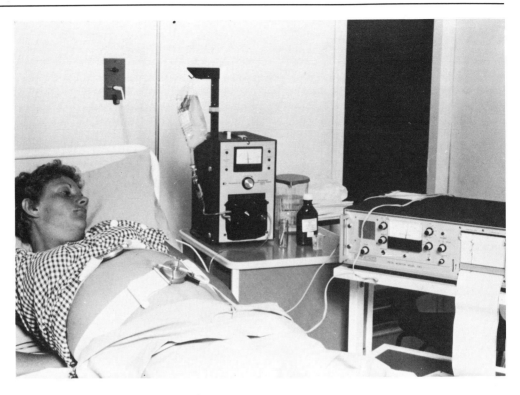

considered at greater risk of dying – because the woman has ★high blood pressure or ★diabetes, for example – are monitored by a cardiotocograph (CTG) once each week, and sometimes more often. The test is painless and takes about 20 minutes.

In labour, a fetal heart monitor may be used in every case, or only for women who are believed to be at special risk of losing the baby. Many obstetricians are divided over

The fetal heart monitor is an electronic machine that picks up the heartbeats of the baby

the usefulness of monitoring every labour. It is probably unnecessary to monitor every labour, and some women who have been monitored object to the procedure. They dislike being linked to a machine by wires, and feel that monitoring distorts the normal progress of childbirth.

Fetal maturity

As pregnancy progresses, the fetus grows and becomes more mature. If the woman knows the date of her last menstrual period and has been examined in the first 10 weeks of pregnancy, the clinical estimation of fetal maturity is highly accurate. A high degree of accuracy can also be obtained by making an ★ultrasound picture of the fetus at about 12 weeks or about 20 weeks. However, some women do not seek ★antenatal care until late in pregnancy, when ultrasound, although helpful, is less accurate for estimating fetal

maturity. In these cases it is more difficult to determine the maturity of the fetus. This is not especially important unless the baby needs to be delivered because the mother has developed ★high blood pressure, or has ★diabetes, or the pregnancy has advanced beyond term. In these circumstances the baby may die in the uterus and be stillborn, or alternatively, be delivered unexpectedly immature after ★induction of labour.

The most important body system for a baby as regards survival is its respiratory system, because it has to be able to breathe easily. The maturity of the fetal lungs can be determined by taking a sample of amniotic fluid by *amniocentesis and measuring certain substances in it. Two tests are currently used. The L:S ratio depends on the amount of the substances lethicin and sphingomyelin in the amniotic fluid. As pregnancy advances, the amount of the former increases more rapidly than the amount of the latter. When there is twice as much lecithin as sphingomyelin in the fluid, it is considered that the baby's lungs are mature, and he is unlikely to have respiratory problems after birth. Another substance, phosphatylglycerol, also increases as pregnancy advances, and its level in the amniotic fluid may be used as an index of the maturity of the baby's lungs. X-rays are no longer used to establish the maturity of the fetus.

Fetal monitoring in pregnancy

One of the purposes of *antenatal care is to monitor the health of the fetus. This is done both by detecting conditions in the mother which might lead to the baby's death, and by monitoring the baby itself. Certain pregnancies carry a higher risk to the baby, such as those complicated by *pre-eclampsia, haemorrhage, *diabetes, or twins. Between 1945 and 1975, the well-being of the fetus was monitored by measuring the level of the hormones oestriol or placental lactogen in the mother's urine or blood. The technique was complicated. With the development of machines like the *fetal heart monitor, physical methods became practicable. Doctors also became aware that the mother could monitor the health of her baby by counting the number of times he moved, or kicked. This has led in many places to the replacement of the hormone tests by physical tests, involving the mother.

In late pregnancy, the fetus moves, or kicks, over 100 times a day and it has been found that if the fetus moves 10 times or more a day, it is healthy and not at extra risk of dying (see *Fetal movements). If the movements fall below 10, the mother should report this to her doctor who will usually arrange for a Non Stress Test. A machine called a cardiotocograph is attached by wires to detecting devices on the woman's abdomen and the fetal heart rate is recorded. If the baby's heart rate increases in response to a uterine contraction or to a stimulus, such as palpation, the test is said to be 'reactive', and the baby is presumed to be at no increased risk. A 'non-reactive' response requires action; this may involve further tests, or the doctor may recommend that the baby should be delivered either by *induction of labour or by a *Caesarean section.

In many clinics, every mother records the Fetal Kick Count several times a week, or each day. Studies have shown that this technique, together with the Non Stress Test, has reduced the possibility of a fetus dying in the uterus, as measures are taken to deliver it in cases of risk.

Fetal movements

The fetus makes movements from about the 8th week of pregnancy, but the mother is not able to detect them until the 16th week. At first she feels fluttering movements, when the baby is said to have 'quickened'. This used to be a matter of some importance in previous centuries, because once quickening had occurred the fetus was considered to be alive and a pregnant woman could not be hanged for murder until after childbirth.

Fetal movements, which are felt as kicks, continue throughout pregnancy, reaching a peak at the 32nd week when over 100 movements occur each day. After this the frequency falls to about 80 movements a day at 40 weeks. Using electronic methods it has been established that women detect over 85 per cent of the movements made by the fetus. Fetal movements are most frequent in the evening but occur throughout the day (and sometimes during the night, waking the mother). There is a wide variation in the pattern of fetal movements. Some fetuses sleep during the day and are active in the evening, others have the opposite pattern.

Recent research has shown the value of counting fetal movements as an indicator of fetal well-being (Fetal Kick Count). Usually the mother is asked to record the number of kicks starting at 9 a.m. until the fetus has kicked 10 times; or she may be asked to record the kicks for an hour in the morning, and if the fetus has not kicked 10 times, to record the kicks for an hour in the afternoon and in the evening. If the mother feels her baby kick more than 10 times during the day, she can be assured that it is healthy. If less than 10 kicks are felt, she should report this to her doctor so that he can arrange for a Non Stress Test (see ★Fetal monitoring).

Fetal positions in pregnancy

During pregnancy the fetus grows and develops in the fluid contained within the ★amniotic sac. The amniotic fluid supports it in an almost weightless condition, which means that it can move about freely. Its movement is reduced in late pregnancy when its size is large compared with the amount of fluid. It is usual for the position of the fetus in the uterus to be checked by the doctor examining the woman's abdomen and palpating it to feel the fetus. If he is in any doubt he may order an ★ultrasound picture to determine the position of the fetus. Up to the 28th week, when there is a relatively large volume of amniotic fluid, it is likely that the fetus will be in a different position at each visit. It may be head down (a cephalic presentation), or with its head in the upper part of the uterus and the buttocks in the lower part (a breech presentation), or it may be cross-ways (a transverse or shoulder presentation). After the 30th week of pregnancy, the great majority of babies settle with their head over the mother's pelvis, and their buttocks in the wider, upper part of the uterus. By the 40th week, 96 per cent of babies lie in this position, as cephalic presentation, and between 3 and 4 per cent lie as breech presentation. In some cases the back of the baby is on the right side of the uterus, and in others on the left. By gently palpating the uterus, the doctor can determine whether the fetus is lying as a cephalic or a breech presentation. This is of some importance at about the 34th week, as the doctor may wish to try to turn a breech baby into a cephalic presentation with head down. The various fetal positions are illustrated in the drawings on page 88.

Fetoscopy

The fetoscope is a system of lenses placed in a narrow needle, which is only 2 mm in diameter. The instrument is introduced through the abdomen and the uterus so that its tip lies in the ★amniotic sac. This permits the doctor to look at the fetus and obtain a sample of its blood or, rarely, its skin. Originally, the fetoscope was used to look for congenital abnormalities of the fetus, but has been superseded by ★ultrasound for this purpose. Its principal use is to obtain samples of fetal blood in the investigation of ★thalassaemia (Mediterranean anaemia). The procedure is called fetoscopy. Fetoscopy is usually made at about the 16th to 18th week of pregnancy,

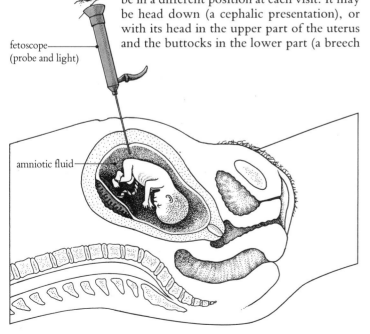

fetoscope
(probe and light)

amniotic fluid

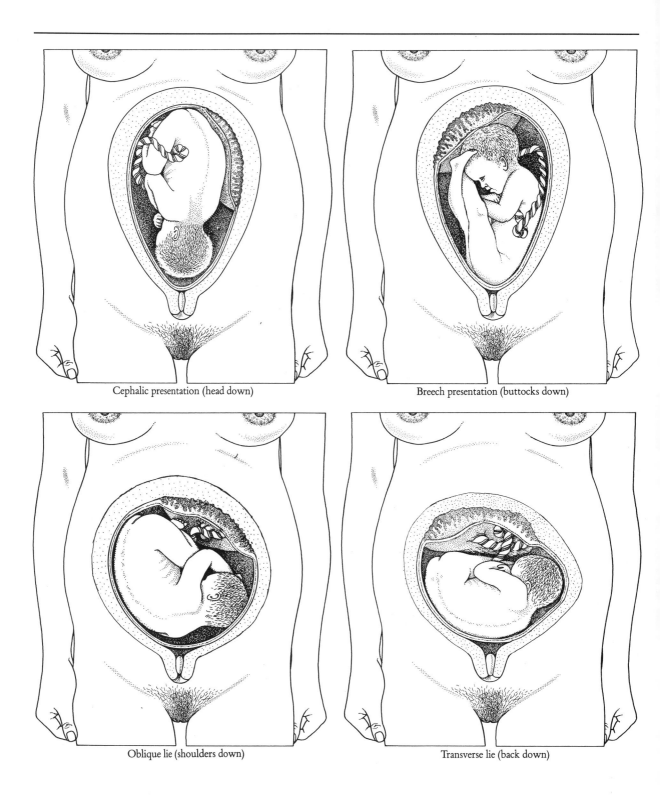

Cephalic presentation (head down)

Breech presentation (buttocks down)

Oblique lie (shoulders down)

Transverse lie (back down)

after ultrasound has detected where the placenta is situated. In the few centres where fetoscopy is carried out, the procedure is made under ultrasonic vision, until the needle lies inside the amniotic sac. The needle is then moved until it punctures a blood vessel in the umbilical cord adjacent to the placenta, and a sample of blood is taken.

Fetus

Fetus (also spelt foetus) is the name given to the growing baby (called an *embryo) from the time all its major organs and structures have been formed (by about the 50th day of pregnancy) to the time it is born, when it is called a neonate. The growth of the fetus in the uterus is dramatic. By the 60th day (8½ weeks) after the last menstrual period it is 30 mm long; four weeks later it is 90 mm long and weighs 14 g. By the 20th week of pregnancy it is 250 mm long and weighs 300 g. When the pregnancy has reached 40 weeks, or 'full term', the fetus is 500 mm long and weighs about 3300 g.

Fibroids

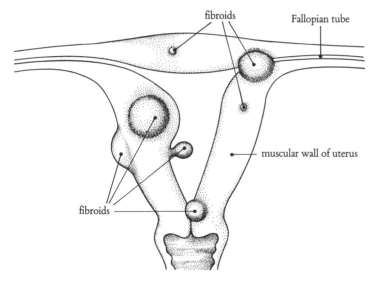

fibroids

Fallopian tube

muscular wall of uterus

fibroids

About one woman in 5 is said to develop one or more fibroids in her uterus by the time she is in her forties. A fibroid (or myoma) is a benign tumour of muscle which develops in the muscular wall of the uterus. The fibroid starts as a tiny pea-sized growth, and may develop over a number of years to form a lump the size of an orange or even larger. In most cases several fibroids of varying sizes grow together. Fibroids usually cause no symptoms, unless they distort the cavity of the uterus when heavy or irregular menstruation may occur, often associated with blood clots and cramp-like pains. Large fibroids may exert pressure on the bladder, causing discomfort or frequency of urination, or on the bowel, when backache or constipation may occur. The doctor makes the diagnosis by examining the woman's pelvis, and sometimes ordering an *ultrasound picture. Treatment depends on the age of the woman, on her desire for children, and on the size and position of the fibroids. Small fibroids which cause no symptoms require no treatment, unless they distort the cavity of the uterus and cause infertility. If a woman desires children, the fibroids can be 'shelled' out of the uterus, and the shape of the uterus restored to normal, by an operation called myomectomy. *Hysterectomy may be advised if a woman has had her family and the fibroids are causing symptoms.

Fontanelle

The skull of a fetus is soft, as the bones are separated from each other and enclosed in a membrane called the periosteum. This arrangement enables the skull bones to move without damage during childbirth and the baby's head to grow quickly after birth. The

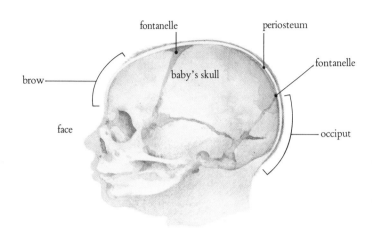

areas of the skull where only membrane covers the underlying brain are called sutures, and the wide area where three or four skull bones meet is called a fontanelle. The main, or 'anterior', fontanelle can be felt on top of the baby's head and is often referred to as the 'soft spot'. It can often be seen to pulsate, especially when the baby is crying or has a fever. Many mothers are reluctant to touch the area for fear of hurting the baby. However, the membranes and skin which cover the fontanelle are extremely tough and protective. The fontanelle gradually gets smaller as the baby's skull grows, and by the time the baby is between 12 and 18 months old the fontanelle has closed completely.

Forceps, obstetrical

The first obstetrical forceps was invented by the Chamberlen family 400 years ago, and kept a secret for nearly a century. Today the obstetrical forceps is a precision-made

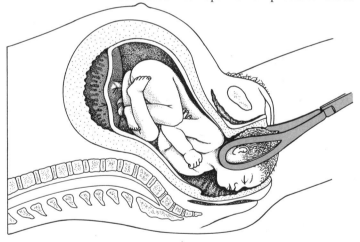

instrument which is used if progress in childbirth is delayed, when it is carefully applied to the baby's head in the mother's vagina. Before the obstetrical forceps is introduced, the woman is given a local anaesthetic, an *epidural anaesthetic, or, occasionally, a general anaesthetic. Forceps are sometimes referred to as 'tongs', but unlike tongs, obstetrical forceps consist of two entirely separate parts, which are locked together when they have been introduced into the vagina, one on each side of the baby's head. When the uterus contracts, the doctor pulls on the handles of the forceps and helps the baby's head emerge from the vagina. The number of women who are delivered by forceps varies, depending on the current medical practice, the doctor's choice, and, occasionally, the mother's preference. In Britain, about one baby in 5 is delivered by forceps.

Frigidity

'Frigid' is the word used by some men to describe a woman who is sexually unresponsive or who fails to reach orgasm with the particular man in the way and at the time he desires. Women are not frigid. What has actually occurred is that the couple do not have a close sexual relationship and the woman feels embarrassed and unable to talk with the man about ways in which he can help her to become sexually aroused. In place of the term 'frigidity', other, more appropriate and sympathetic words should be used in these circumstances to describe the woman's *sexual problems.

G

Galactorrhoea

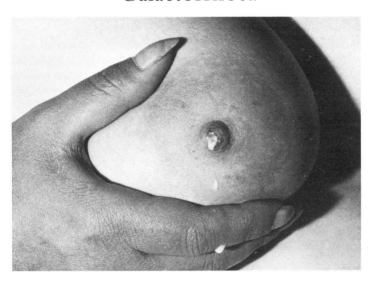

Galactorrhoea is the inappropriate secretion of breast milk by a woman who is not pregnant or breast-feeding (lactating). Lactation depends mainly on the secretion of the pituitary gland hormone ★prolactin, and the presence of galactorrhoea usually implies that excessive quantities of the hormone are being secreted. Excessive secretion of prolactin may be due to a small tumour of the pituitary gland, or may occur because the woman is taking certain medications. If galactorrhoea persists for more than 4 weeks, and particularly if it is associated with ★amenorrhoea, investigations are required, and any necessary treatment started. The investigations usually include a careful history, an X-ray picture of the skull, and the measurement of certain hormones in a blood sample.

Genital crisis

A small number of female babies develop a bloody discharge from their vagina, and may develop some degree of swelling of the external genitals during the first few days after birth. This is called the 'genital crisis'. When the baby is in the uterus, the hormone oestrogen produced by the mother enters its blood and stimulates the lining of its uterus to a modest degree. After birth, the supply of oestrogen is withdrawn (because the baby is now an individual) and as it is no longer stimulated, the lining of the uterus crumbles, producing a small menstrual period. After this the lining rapidly heals. The girl will not menstruate again until her own sex hormones, produced after ★puberty, stimulate the uterus. The condition is normal and no treatment is needed.

Genital herpes

Infection of the genital area by the herpes virus *(Herpes genitalis)* is becoming increasingly common in women and men. More women than men are infected as a woman's genital area is warmer and moister than a man's penis. Genital herpes resembles the herpes which causes cold sores on the mouth, but the viruses are not identical. Type 1 virus usually causes cold sores, type 2 virus usually causes genital herpes.

The infection is transmitted sexually and the virus enters the skin through an invisible abrasion. Once inside the skin it multiplies and causes an itching or burning sensation.

Small blisters appear which develop into painful ulcers, and the surrounding tissues may become swollen and painful. The ulcers heal in 7 to 10 days and disappear. In between 2 and 5 per cent of women the virus persists in the nerves which supply the genitals. It may be dormant for weeks or months, when for some reason it is reactivated and the herpes infection recurs.

There is no specific treatment, as all the medications which have been used have proved ineffective. All that can be done until the ulcers heal is to take analgesic tablets, and to paint the ulcers with gentian violet or use

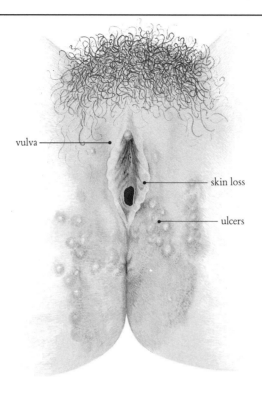

vulva

skin loss

ulcers

an analgesic cream. In the past two years, a drug called acyclovir has been under investigation for the treatment of initial severe attacks of herpes. Acyclovir is most effective if given by intravenous injection; but when taken by mouth or applied to the herpes ulcers it is reported to reduce the pain and duration of the infection. Unfortunately, acyclovir does not seem to help in recurrent herpes infections.

As herpes is sexually transmitted and contagious, any person (male or female) who develops herpes ulcers should avoid sexual intercourse until they have healed completely. If a pregnant woman develops genital herpes or has a recurrence in the last 10 weeks of pregnancy, swabs are taken periodically from her cervix. If the swab grows herpes virus on culture in the last 4 weeks of pregnancy, the baby is delivered by ★Caesarean section, as herpes can be transmitted to the baby from the genital tract of the mother. The infection may result in severe illness or even the death of the baby.

Genital warts

Increasing numbers of both women and men are suffering from genital warts (*condylomata acuminata*, or 'sharp-ended knobs'). The warts, which are caused by a virus and spread by sexual contact, vary in size from a pinhead to large cauliflower-like growths. In women, they prefer to grow in the warm, moist areas of the perineum, the inside of the labia majora or the labia minora, or in the vagina. The virus may be a factor in producing cancer of the cervix, so for this reason, and also because the warts are contagious, they should be treated.

Treatment is to touch each wart on the vulva with podophyllin. This is a caustic substance, so the unaffected skin is protected with a jelly. The podophyllin is allowed to dry and then left for 2 hours, after which the woman should wash her vulva thoroughly with water. The treatment is repeated weekly until the wart disappears. Podophyllin cannot be used on vaginal warts as it may cause burning, nor should it be used during pregnancy. The treatment of vaginal warts is

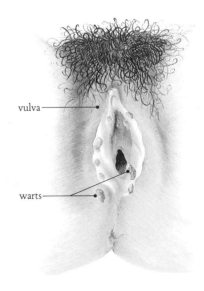

vulva

warts

to freeze them with a small instrument (cryosurgery) or to burn them (with an electric cautery).

Gestagens

Gestagens (progestogens, progestins) are a group of chemical substances which act on the cells and tissues of the body in ways which are similar to the natural hormone *progesterone. In general, they regulate the way in which *oestrogen stimulates the cells of the genital tract and breasts to develop and to divide. The drugs have proved useful in reducing the menstrual loss of women who have *menstrual problems, particularly heavy menstruation. Gestagens are used in the contraceptive *pill, where they add to the effect of oestrogen in preventing pregnancy and regulate the 'period' which occurs each month. They are also used alone in other forms of contraception, as the *Mini-pill or *injectable contraceptives. The drugs have been used to treat *premenstrual tension, though with limited success. Gestagens are useful in treating the symptoms of the *menopause, and are usually given for about 10 days each month. They are also used to prevent the development of cancer of the lining of the uterus (*endometrial cancer). Large doses of gestagens, given by injection, have also been used to control inoperable endometrial cancer, with some success.

The gestagens commonly available are hydroxyprogesterone (Proluton-Depot), norethisterone (Primolut-N, Micronor), levonorgestrel (Duoluton, Microlut, Microval), dydrogesterone (Duphaston), and medroxyprogesterone (Provera and Depo-Provera).

Glucose tolerance test

In pregnancy a delay occurs in the transfer of the glucose from the mother's blood to her tissues. This results in a higher level of blood sugar, and provides the fetus with a more readily available supply of energy. The raised blood sugar level often leads to the appearance of sugar in the mother's urine. In about 2 per cent of women, the 'glucose intolerance' – the delayed transfer of glucose to the tissues – is more severe, and the woman is said to have *gestational diabetes. This condition adds a slightly increased risk to the fetus, if the woman is aged 25 or over.

For this reason many obstetric units now screen all pregnant women for gestational diabetes, either by taking a sample of blood and measuring its level of glucose, or by asking the woman to drink a sweetened orange drink (containing 50 g of glucose) and measuring the glucose level of a blood sample taken one hour later. If the blood level of glucose exceeds a certain amount (7.6 mmol/litre), then a glucose tolerance test is performed. The woman eats a normal diet for 3 days, fasts for 12 hours, and rests for half an hour before the test. She is given a glucose drink, and samples of blood are taken at 30-minute intervals for 2 or 3 hours. The diagnosis of gestational diabetes is made or excluded by studying the results of the test.

Gonorrhoea

Gonorrhoea is a sexually transmitted disease and is usually spread from person to person by sexual intercourse, although it can infect people during oral or anal sex, or, rarely, a newborn baby's eyes may be infected by its mother during childbirth.

During sexual intercourse, the glands of the cervix, or the urethra, may be infected. Three to seven days after contact, the woman notices that it is painful to urinate, and a discharge may seep from her urethra, or from her vagina. The symptoms may be severe, or so mild that they are not noticed. Mild symptoms occur in about half of women infected, who are then likely to infect their next sexual partner. If the woman is not treated, the infection may spread into her uterus and infect the Fallopian tubes, causing pelvic infection and possible sterility. Gonorrhoea is cured by penicillin, given in

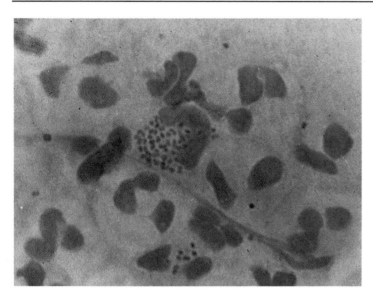

conjunction with another drug, to keep the blood level of penicillin high. As 50 per cent of women who are infected are unaware that they have the disease, it is recommended that any woman who has multiple partners should be checked for gonorrhoea every six months or so. This is done by laboratory examination of swabs taken from her urethra and cervix.

Gonorrhoea is caused by the bacterium, Neisseria gonorrhoeae, as seen here through a microscope

Grande multipara

This term was given over half a century ago by an Irish obstetrician to a woman who had given birth to five children and was currently embarked on her sixth pregnancy. It used to be the case that grande multiparae were more likely to develop ★high blood pressure or ★diabetes in pregnancy and to have a difficult labour. Today with improved methods of family planning fewer women fall into this category; and with improved obstetric care, the problems have been considerably reduced.

Granuloma inguinale

Granuloma inguinale is a sexually transmitted disease which is caused by a small bacillus. It is uncommon in temperate climates but occurs more frequently in the tropics. Between 3 days and 3 months of being infected the woman develops multiple small, irregularly shaped ulcers on the inner surface of the small lips of her vulva or in the entrance to her vagina. The ulcers tend to spread, unless treated, and if they become infected are painful and itchy. If this happens the woman's external genitals may become massively swollen. Fortunately, however, the disease responds quickly to prescribed antibiotics and leaves no scarring provided it is treated early enough.

H

Haematoma, pelvic

A haematoma is a collection of blood in the pelvis, which is usually clotted, and occurs following injury, an *ectopic pregnancy, or gynaecological surgery. In its early stages it may be painful and analgesics may be required. After a while, the pain goes and the haematoma is slowly absorbed, a process which may take a few weeks. Occasionally, bleeding continues and the pelvic haematoma increases in size. The woman develops increasing pain, deep in her pelvis, and may notice a lump in her abdomen. If the bleeding continues surgery is needed to remove the clotted blood and also to place a ligature around the blood vessel which is responsible for the bleeding.

Haemorrhoids

Haemorrhoids (or piles) are essentially varicose veins of the anus. Like varicose veins in other parts of the body, they tend to occur in families (which suggests a hereditary factor), and they are similarly caused by pressure which hinders the return of blood. They are aggravated by straining to evacuate chronically constipated motions. They are common in late pregnancy, and after childbirth, when the enlarged uterus prevents the free return of blood from the veins of the lower bowel.

There are two kinds of haemorrhoids: internal and external. *Internal haemorrhoids* are the more common type, and often they cause no trouble apart from slight bleeding during a bowel motion. In other cases they prolapse (slip down) outside the anus during straining, and can be pushed in again. They may later prolapse at any time, when they cause discomfort; this can be relieved by ointments. Occasionally an 'attack of piles' occurs; blood congests the prolapsed haemorrhoid and it is unable to return, with the result that it becomes swollen, painful, and inflamed. If it is left, the blood will clot, causing a 'thrombosed pile'. In cases of permanently prolapsed haemorrhoids, treatment is usually desirable. Three methods are available. The first is to stretch the anus widely (under an anaesthetic). The second is to inject a substance which will fix the mucous membrane covering the pile to the underlying muscle, to prevent it prolapsing. A recent advance is to use an infra-red coagulator which is quick and painless. The third method is to excise the pile surgically.

External haemorrhoids may be found alone or in conjunction with internal haemorrhoids. They cause few problems unless a clot occurs, when a painful swelling appears at the margin of the anus. In most cases it subsides after a few days, but surgery can be used to relieve the pain if it is excessive.

Hairiness

The amount of body hair a woman has depends to some extent on her ethnic origin. Chinese women, for example, have relatively little body hair, while some Southern European women have much more. When the amount of body hair, or its growth on certain parts of the body such as the face or legs, is excessive compared with others in the same ethnic group, the condition is called hirsutism.

Hirsute women are frequently disturbed about their *body-image and feel that they are less attractive than women who do not have a lot of body hair. If a hirsute woman has signs of *virilism, as shown by an enlarged clitoris, a deepening voice, the lack of menstruation, or receding hair, then the condition requires careful investigation. However, most hirsute women have none of these signs, and their hairiness is due to an increased secretion into their blood and tissues of the male hormone testosterone, or alternatively to an increased sensitivity to this hormone which is normally present in the blood in small amounts. The blood level of testosterone can be measured quite easily and the diagnosis confirmed.

Most hirsute women wish to have body hair reduced and several methods are available. Cosmetic aids such as shaving (which, contrary to popular belief, does not cause increased hair growth), bleaching, waxing, depilatory creams, and electrolysis often help. Electrolysis is expensive, may be painful, and should only be used if the excess hair is coarse and sparse. It should only be carried out by an expert.

Drugs may help, but these must be prescribed with care. Some hairy women notice an improvement if they take a sequential contraceptive (see *Pill). More recently a drug called cyproterone acetate has been used to treat hairiness. Cyproterone is a drug which prevents testosterone being taken up by the hair follicles and may also reduce its secretion. It is given for 10 days of the menstrual cycle, starting on day 5, and at the same time small doses of *oestrogen are given and are continued for a further 10 days to keep the menstrual cycle regular. Treatment must continue for at least 3 months before there is any reduction in the hirsutism, and usually the drugs have to be continued for 9 months to obtain the maximum response. One woman in every 5 using cyproterone reports the side-effect of tiredness, and a similar proportion find they put on weight. One woman in 10 complains of a reduction in sexual arousal. However, as 4 women in 5 obtain considerable reduction in body hair, most consider the side-effects of the drug acceptable.

Heartburn

Heartburn is not uncommon during late pregnancy and may occur at other times. The cause is a relaxation of the muscular valve which guards the junction between the oesophagus and the stomach. This allows some of the acid stomach contents to regurgitate into the lower oesophagus and to irritate it. Treatment for this condition is to eat small meals often, to avoid spicy foods, to stop smoking, and to use antacid tablets or mixtures as necessary in order to relieve the discomfort.

Heart disease and pregnancy

During pregnancy the heart has to work harder to move an increased volume of blood at a faster rate through the blood vessels. It does this by beating faster and by ejecting a larger amount of blood each time it beats. The additional strain on the heart begins at the 8th week of pregnancy and reaches a maximum at the 30th week.

If a woman has heart disease – and this affects about one woman in every 200 to 400 – pregnancy imposes an extra strain on the damaged heart. Provided the woman seeks *antenatal care early and follows instructions, no harm should come to her or her baby. She will need to be seen by her doctor at regular intervals when he will listen to her heart and lungs and check her pulse rate. She will be asked to report if she becomes breathless, especially at night; if she is excessively tired or develops a cough. Her blood will be examined and she may be required to take iron tablets to avoid *anaemia. Her weight gain will be regulated. Depending on the severity of the heart disease, the pregnant woman may be asked to relax and take more rest during the day.

The management of childbirth is not very different from that of other women, but *forceps delivery is used more frequently and digitalis (a heart strengthening drug) may be needed if the woman's heart shows strain during labour. During or after childbirth she may be given antibiotics to prevent infection, although not all physicians agree that this is necessary. After childbirth the burden on the mother's heart continues and she is closely observed for the first 24 hours to make sure heart failure does not occur.

Hepatitis

Viral infections of the liver are caused by three different viruses, designated hepatitis A virus (HAV), hepatitis B virus (HBV), and hepatitis non A-non B. Hepatitis A is usually a mild infection accompanied by nausea, lack of appetite, and later by a swollen liver and jaundice. Similar symptoms occur following infection with hepatitis B virus but the disease is more serious and may cause chronic liver damage.

Infection by hepatitis B virus is relatively uncommon among white adults (varying from 0.3 to 1.0 per cent) but is much more common in Asian and Pacific Islanders when it affects up to 20 per cent of adults. It is also more common among white adults who have liver disease, who are drug addicts, who work in a renal dialysis unit or handle blood, or those who are sexually promiscuous.

HBV infection may be transmitted during childbirth to the baby or to the medical attendants. It is recommended that when a large number of Asian women or other women in the higher risk category are cared for in pregnancy, a blood test is made to measure hepatitis B surface antigen (HBsAg) which identifies those women infected with the virus. If HBsAg is found it means the woman either has had hepatitis B infection during pregnancy or is a carrier. During childbirth the attendants must take care not to contaminate their eyes, mouth, or any cut with the woman's blood, and the baby is given an injection of hepatitis B immune globulin within 24 hours of birth, to prevent it being infected. A vaccine to protect those who come into contact with those who have HBV has now been developed.

High-risk pregnancy

This rather loose term is used to identify those pregnancies in which the mother is at greater risk of losing the baby, which is either stillborn or is born prematurely and dies in the first month of life. Women who come into the 'high-risk' category require increased attention during pregnancy so that measures may be taken which will rescue the baby from a hostile environment within the uterus. The main causes of higher risk are listed opposite.

If a woman is in one of these groups, she will be checked at frequent intervals throughout her pregnancy. She may be asked to monitor her baby's well-being by counting its movements (*Fetal Kick Count), or other methods of *fetal monitoring may be used, such as *cardiotocography and *ultrasound examinations. If the tests show the baby is under an increasing risk of

dying, the pregnancy may be terminated by *Caesarean section or by *induction of labour.

(1) The development of *high blood pressure in pregnancy (also called *pre-eclampsia, toxaemia, and pregnancy-induced hypertension).

(2) Diseases such as *diabetes, *anaemia, *heart disease, and hypertension, which preceded the pregnancy.

(3) Pregnancy which has lasted for more than 2 weeks beyond the expected date ('prolonged pregnancy').

(4) *Multiple pregnancy.

(5) *Rhesus iso-immune disease.

(6) Pregnancy in which the fetus is not growing appropriately ('fetal growth retardation').

Home birth

In most developed countries over 95 per cent of births take place in hospital. The exception is Holland where half the number of babies

are born at home. There has recently been a demand for home birth, its proponents observing that as women are healthier today, have better nutritional standards, and can be screened more efficiently during pregnancy, those women who are at low risk of developing problems could safely deliver at home. They also note the very low rate of *perinatal mortality in Holland, which indicates that nowadays home birth is relatively safe. Those women who have delivered at home tell of the exhilarating experience of giving birth supported by their family, in familiar surroundings, where the woman feels she has control over her body. They compare this with the experience of giving birth in hospital, in a busy, rather regimented, clinical and impersonal environment governed by regulations.

Home birth may have a place in modern obstetric care, but most doctors are concerned that the danger to the baby is increased in home birth. During labour the baby may develop 'distress' (see *Fetal distress), indicating that action is needed to deliver him, or after birth he may not be able to breathe properly. In a hospital, the facilities are available to deal quickly with both of these conditions, which may not be possible at home. Occasionally, a woman may bleed excessively after the birth (*postpartum haemorrhage); again, in hospital this can be dealt with immediately, but in the home problems may arise which can place the woman at risk.

The dangers to the baby and the risk of postpartum haemorrhage were the main reasons why, over the past twenty years, home birth has been replaced by hospital birth. The experience being obtained in *Birth Centres will help doctors evaluate if home birth can be offered to women as a safe choice in childbirth.

Homosexuality

A homosexual woman is one whose emotional and sexual needs can only be fully satisfied by another woman. She forms a relationship with a woman in preference to a man, in many cases having first lived with, or been married to, a man, and often having given birth to a child or children. The new relationship usually, but not always, includes *sexual pleasuring.

There is no convincing evidence that homosexuality is inherited, or due to a genetic defect, or caused by a hormonal 'imbalance', or that the woman has been seduced by an older homosexual. Homosexual women are neither sick, nor are they criminals, nor are they sinful. Apart from their erotic preference, their behaviour, their mental stability, their physical health, and their attitudes are similar to those of heterosexual women.

Most lesbians are not identifiable in the community. They look and behave like other women. Only a small minority – probably less than 5 per cent of all homosexual women – conform to the 'butch' stereotype of an aggressive, male-looking woman; or to the 'fem' stereotype of a passive, dependent, soft woman.

In their relationships, lesbians are no more and no less promiscuous or permissive than heterosexual women: most of their relationships are stable and last for a long period. Homosexual women use many of the same behaviours as heterosexual women to express their love and sexual desire. They cuddle, kiss, fondle, and stimulate each other's breasts and bodies, often for longer periods and with greater mutual pleasure than occurs in many heterosexual relationships, as they are less inhibited in telling each other what gives them most pleasure.

Most lesbians are able to reach orgasm through masturbation; by having their clitoral area digitally stimulated by their partner, by body-to-body friction, especially of the lower abdomen and pubic area (tribadism) or by cunnilingus (*oral sex). In contrast to heterosexual relationships, when cunnilingus is often seen by the man as a necessary step to get the woman ready for sexual intercourse, cunnilingus between lesbians is more sensitive and imaginative, and is shared and enjoyed by both partners. Contrary to popular belief (mainly of men), very few lesbians use a *dildo or an 'artificial penis' in order to reach orgasm.

Lesbians face several problems in society. Although many homosexuals are now able to 'come out' and announce that they are gay, others find this a threat and continue to conceal their homosexuality because of the fear of discrimination. This discrimination exists, and may engender feelings of guilt. These feelings may be marked if the lesbian is a Christian, as the Churches have a poor record of helping homosexuals.

Lesbians who have children from a previous heterosexual relationship, or who are in a homosexual relationship and want children, face problems as both society and the law place many barriers in their way. A woman whose marriage is dissolved because of her homosexuality may be refused custody of her child. A woman wishing to have a child in a homosexual relationship must either find an appropriate male for sexual intercourse (which she may find distasteful) or seek *artificial insemination (AID). Many doctors refuse to carry out artificial insemination for lesbians, and permission to adopt a child is rarely granted. The antipathy of society is based on the false belief that a child brought up by a lesbian couple will either suffer psychologically or will be harmed physically. The small amount of scientific evidence which is available (as opposed to anecdotal polemics) shows that children brought up by homosexual couples are psycho-sexually normal, are well cared for, and much loved.

Hormone replacement therapy

The concept of hormone replacement therapy (HRT) was introduced in the 1960s. It is based on the fact that after the *menopause, the quantity of the female sex hormone *oestrogen circulating in a woman's blood is dramatically reduced. Proponents of HRT believe that the lack of oestrogen increases certain body changes such as dry hair, wrinkling of the skin, sexual problems (such as dry vagina), and *osteoporosis. Oestrogen deficiency is also thought to cause some mental degenerative changes such as depression, irritability, and loss of memory. Those in support of HRT say that all the changes can be prevented by giving oestrogen continuously to every woman from the time of her menopause into old age. They argue further that women have a *right* to HRT, for two reasons. The first is that, biologically, a woman is the only female animal whose reproductive function (and hence sex-hormonal function) ceases many years before she dies. The second is that because of improved nutrition, public health, and hygiene, many more women now survive to old age. About 10 per cent of women are over 65 in developed countries. It is claimed that to deprive them of hormone therapy is to condemn them prematurely to degenerative diseases.

The concept of HRT seemed very attractive and, in the United States particularly, a large proportion of post-menopausal women were prescribed oestrogen in the 1960s and early 1970s which they were to take each day until they died.

Unfortunately, three problems have arisen. First, it has been found that many of the degenerative changes are not related to oestrogen deficiency. Only *hot flushes (with the associated night sweats and insomnia) and a dry, painful vagina seem to be due to a lack of oestrogen in the blood. Second, of the long-term degenerative conditions, only osteoporosis may be delayed by using HRT. Third, the use of oestrogen in HRT has been found to be associated with an increased risk (three- to eight-fold) of developing uterine (*endometrial) cancer. This means that if HRT were accepted by all post-menopausal women, the risk of developing endometrial cancer would rise from one per 1000 women each year to about 6 per 1000 women each year.

With knowledge of these risks, fewer women are now prepared to take oestrogen continuously over a long period of time, and those who do take oestrogen, take it over shorter periods of time, in conjunction with the second sex hormone, progesterone (or, more accurately, its synthetic substitute, *gestagen). Gestagen is used in addition to oestrogen because the combination has been

Hormone replacement therapy
Hot flushes
Hyaline membrane disease

shown to provide protection against endometrial cancer. However, the combination is associated with uterine bleeding which occurs at rather unpredictable intervals and can be disturbing.

The use of HRT has become unfashionable. Even the term HRT was a misnomer, because the oestrogen did not return all the hormone levels to those found before the menopause.

Hot flushes

Hot flushes (or flashes) are a common and annoying accompaniment of the *menopause which affect most women, about one-third of them severely. A hot flush starts as a feeling of heat centred on the face, which spreads to the neck and chest before it disappears after about 2 minutes. Many hot flushes are accompanied or followed by sweating. Investigations have shown that each flush is preceded by a sudden release of luteinizing hormone from the pituitary gland, and the hot flush is accompanied by an increase in the heart rate, a rise in the body temperature, and dilation of the blood vessels in the skin. Hot flushes may occur infrequently or many times a day, and also at night when they may lead to insomnia. They usually start when menstruation ceases at the

menopause, but may begin a year or so earlier. They occur over a period of one to 5 years. If hot flushes are annoying and interfere with a woman's activities, she may be prescribed small amounts of the hormone oestrogen to be taken for 28 days each month, which will relieve the symptoms. The doctor will also prescribe a second hormone (*gestagen) which she takes for the last 10 days of the course. After 7 days of no treatment when a small amount of bleeding, rather like a light menstrual period, may occur, she takes a further course of hormones. Gestagen is given to protect the lining of the uterus (the endometrium) from the stimulating effect of oestrogen, which is associated with cancer (see *Hormone replacement therapy).

Hyaline membrane disease

One of the problems of *preterm birth is that the baby's lungs may not be able to function properly, because they are affected by hyaline membrane disease (HMD). This illness, which is also known as 'respiratory distress syndrome', is due to a lack of a chemical substance called surfactant. Surfactant is formed in the fetal lungs from about the 20th week of pregnancy and the amount present in the lungs increases dramatically between the 32nd and 34th weeks of pregnancy. This substance enables the air sacs which make up the lung to expand easily, filling with air. If it is deficient, the air sacs collapse when the baby breathes out, and it is harder for them to expand when the baby takes in its next breath. Over a few hours the baby finds it increasingly hard to expand his lungs and uses an increased amount of energy trying to breathe. An X-ray of the lungs shows a 'snowstorm pattern' which indicates

the lungs have collapsed air sacs, and hyaline membrane disease is confirmed.

The disease affects between 30 and 50 per cent of babies weighing less than 1500 g at birth, but fewer than 1 per cent of babies weighing more than 2000 g at birth. In the past, one baby in 3 who developed the disease died, but today few babies die. The decline in the number of deaths is due to several factors. It has been found that cortisone encourages the development of surfactant, and an injection of cortisone may be given to mothers threatening to go into labour prematurely if the pregnancy has not reached the end of the 34th week. This reduces the frequency of the disease, but does not eliminate it. Expert care in a Neonatal Care Nursery has reduced the death rate to less than 5 per cent. A new treatment which consists of squirting synthetic surfactant into an affected baby's lungs is currently under trial.

Hysterectomy

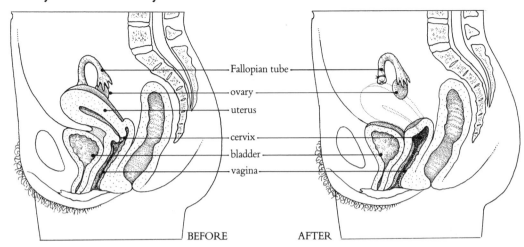

Fallopian tube
ovary
uterus
cervix
bladder
vagina

BEFORE   AFTER

A hysterectomy is an operation to remove the uterus. The frequency with which the operation is performed varies considerably, being higher in Australia and the United States than in Sweden and Britain. This fact suggests that other treatments are available which may be adopted rather than hysterectomy, at least in the first instance. The difference in the frequency of hysterectomy between these countries is probably explained by the fact that in Australia and the United States doctors are more likely to treat some gynaecological conditions by surgery than to prescribe medications, and the patients are more likely to demand a hysterectomy.

A hysterectomy is performed for several reasons:

(**1**) To relieve the symptom of heavy menstrual bleeding which has not responded to hormone treatment.

(**2**) To remove a uterus enlarged by ★fibroids which are causing the symptoms of bleeding, pressure, or pain, or if they enlarge the uterus considerably.

(**3**) As part of an operation to treat ★prolapse.

(**4**) As part of an operation to treat ★endometriosis.

(**5**) As part of an operation to treat ★pelvic infection.

(**6**) To treat ★cancer of the uterus or of the ovaries.

(**7**) Occasionally as a method of sterilization.

The operation is sometimes performed by making a cut into the lower part of the abdomen, and sometimes the uterus is taken out through the vagina. If the woman is undergoing the ★menopause, some doctors also remove the ovaries at the operation, particularly if they are diseased. In all cases the cut vagina is stitched, so that it is much the same size as it was before the operation. When the uterus has been removed, the bowels move to fill the space that would be left. After the operation it is usual for the patient to wake up and find that an intravenous drip is giving her blood or fluid, and this continues for a day or two. If she has had a vaginal hysterectomy, she may also have a catheter in her bladder to allow drainage of urine, and this may be inserted through a tiny cut in the wall of her lower abdomen. As a small leak of bloody serum is usual from her vagina, the patient has to wear a sanitary pad for a few days. She usually goes home after 7 to 10 days and should take things slowly for 2 or 3 weeks, doing a little more each day but resting if she feels tired. If the patient's ovaries were removed before the menopause, she will need to have ★hormone replacement therapy to relieve menopausal symptoms.

The woman can resume sexual intercourse when the cut in the top of the vagina has healed strongly, which takes about 4 weeks, but she can enjoy other forms of ★sexual pleasuring before that if she wishes. In a study of the sexual function of women after hysterectomy about one-third of women were found to enjoy sex more, about one-third enjoyed it less, and in the remaining one-third there was little change. If the woman had a good and satisfying sex life before hysterectomy she was likely to have a good (or a better) sex life after the operation.

Hysterectomy, if done by an experienced surgeon, for a good reason, and after full and frank discussion with the woman, is a satisfactory operation and provides desired relief to most women, who have more energy and are happier. If the operation is done for a trivial reason and without prior discussion, the results are not so good and the dissatisfied women may continue to seek medical, and especially psychiatric, help for unresolved problems, particularly depression. This emphasizes the importance of discussion and counselling before surgery and the need for the woman to have time to think about the operation before it is done, unless cancer is the reason for the hysterectomy. There are several myths about women who have had a hysterectomy: they are all untrue. Hysterectomy does not make a woman become fat; neither does it make her grow hair on her body or face; and furthermore it does not make sex difficult.

Hysterosalpingography

Hysterosalpingography is a method of examining the interior of the uterus and the Fallopian tubes particularly when investigating ★infertility. The examination is carried out in the radiological department of a hospital or clinic. A ★speculum is used to expose the cervix, and a small metal tube is then introduced. The tube is connected to a syringe which is filled with a water-based dye. X-ray pictures are taken as the dye is injected and these appear on a television screen so that both the woman and the doctor can see what is happening. In a fertile woman the dye, which is opaque to X-rays, fills first the uterus and then the Fallopian tubes, and drips from the ends of the tubes into the abdominal cavity. A hysterosalpingogram tells the doctor several things. Firstly, it outlines any distortion in the cavity of the uterus, for example a ★fibroid. Secondly, it shows if the Fallopian tubes are open, or if there is a blockage. Thirdly, it shows where the blockage is, which helps in suggesting treatment.

The procedure is not usually painful but can be occasionally. It can nearly always be done without an anaesthetic. It takes about 5 minutes, and when it is completed the tube is withdrawn from the cervix. The woman may have to have a further X-ray taken of her abdomen, an hour later, but on this occasion nothing is introduced into her vagina. The water-based dye is quickly absorbed from the abdominal cavity and does not have any harmful effect.

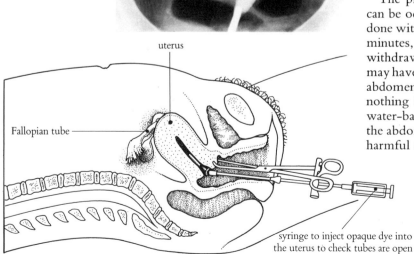

uterus

Fallopian tube

syringe to inject opaque dye into the uterus to check tubes are open

Incest

Incest means sexual activity between members of the same family, and this is usually defined as including uncles, aunts, and grandparents as well as the immediate members. The sexual activity may include fondling, caressing, *masturbation, and *oral sex, as well as *sexual intercourse. Incest occurs much more commonly than is believed, and studies show that between 5 and 10 per cent of the female population have had an incestuous experience. Most remain unreported. The most common form of incest is between brother and sister, the next most common between father and daughter. The incestuous experiences usually occur at intervals over a period of time, and if an adult is involved, the adult initiates the first act. The effect of incest on a child is uncertain, but most reports indicate that incest is emotionally damaging (in the United States, more than half of adolescent prostitutes claim to have been subjected to incest). It is unclear how long the person will remain emotionally disturbed, but those people who are able to receive help and to talk about their feelings to a trained therapist recover more easily. The causes which lead to incest are unknown, as it occurs in all classes of society. Poor family relationships, overcrowding in the home, the influence of alcohol, and drugs may all be involved: but little is known, and intervention impossible. All that can be done is to provide help, support, and comfort for the victims who report incest.

Incompetent cervix

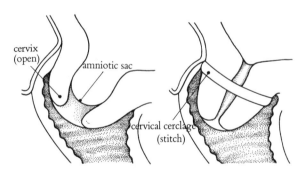

cervix (open)

amniotic sac

cervical cerclage (stitch)

A proportion of women who have a *spontaneous abortion between the 12th and 19th week of pregnancy, or who give birth between the 20th and 29th week, have an 'incompetent cervix'. In this condition, the *cervix is weak and stretches as a result of the pressure of the fetus. As the cervix of the woman stretches and opens, it causes the uterus to contract, which in turn starts an abortion or premature labour.

An incompetent cervix is diagnosed firstly, if the woman has had two or more late abortions or very premature births; secondly, if an examination when she is not pregnant shows that her cervix is weak; thirdly, during pregnancy, if the cervix becomes stretched and this is detected by a vaginal examination.

The treatment is to stitch up the cervix using a wide 'ribbon' and to tie it, rather like tying a string around the neck of a balloon. This stitch, called cervical cerclage, prevents labour from starting, often until the pregnancy is at or near full term. When labour is established, the stitch is cut and the baby is born rapidly. In a few cases, where the woman has had several late abortions, the doctor may suggest a *Caesarean section to avoid the possible hazard of a vaginal birth.

Induction of labour

Induction of labour means that the onset of labour is stimulated artificially instead of waiting for it to start spontaneously. The main reasons for inducing labour are first, conditions of the mother such as *high blood pressure, *antepartum haemorrhage (bleeding before the onset of labour), or prolonged pregnancy; second, conditions of the fetus

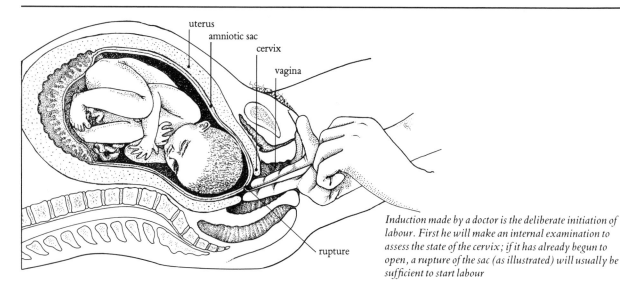

uterus
amniotic sac
cervix
vagina
rupture

Induction made by a doctor is the deliberate initiation of labour. First he will make an internal examination to assess the state of the cervix; if it has already begun to open, a rupture of the sac (as illustrated) will usually be sufficient to start labour

such as a congenital abnormality; third, occasionally labour is induced for social reasons, the so-called 'elective induction' because it is convenient for the woman or her doctor that the baby should be born on a particular date. Elective induction used to be performed in about 40 per cent of all childbirths, but the figure has declined to below 10 per cent in the past ten years, partly because of a change in fashion and partly because elective induction was followed by a higher number of ★Caesarean sections, a higher rate of ★forceps delivery, and more cases of ★jaundice in the baby.

Labour can be induced in several ways, depending on the texture of the cervix and how far it has opened (dilated). If the cervix is soft and at least 2 cm dilated it is said to be 'ripe', and labour can be started by breaking

the waters with a small plastic instrument and following this immediately, or some hours later, with an intravenous drip of ★oxytocin, which encourages the uterus to start contracting.

If the cervix is not 'ripe', in other words if it is firm and not dilated, labour may be induced by a hormone called ★prostaglandin. The prostaglandin is mixed in a thick jelly and is injected into the cervix or is placed in the upper vagina, or may be given in the form of vaginal pessaries or tablets. The procedure may have to be repeated in 2 to 4 hours, until labour is established. Following induction, labour usually begins within 4 to 12 hours, and the woman may usually expect her baby to be born by evening, if labour has been induced in the morning.

Infertility, immunological factors

In a small proportion of infertile couples, where no obvious cause for the infertility can be found, it is possible that spermatozoa are unable to penetrate the cervix because the woman produces antibodies which immobilize or kill them, or, alternatively, that the man himself makes antibodies which damage his own sperms before they are ejaculated. Several tests have been proposed to identify these immunological factors in infertility. Most consist of taking a sample of

sperm and mixing it with blood serum from the woman. If the sperms become immobile (stop 'shaking'), the test is considered positive. However, positive tests have been found in women who became pregnant, so it has been uncertain what the tests meant.

A recent test measures anti-sperm antibody, which appears to be more accurate in identifying the problem. In a study in the United States of over 600 infertile patients, where no cause had been found, anti-sperm antibodies were detected in the blood plasma of 13 per cent of the women and 7 per cent of the men. Further studies will show if this small group of infertile patients can be helped to achieve a pregnancy by giving the affected partner the drug cortisone over a period of 21 days. An alternative method is to bypass the cervical immunological block by artificially inseminating the sperm into the woman's uterus at the time of *ovulation.

Infertility, investigations

A couple who have been trying to achieve a pregnancy for a year, and have failed to do so, can be considered infertile, and may seek help. For a woman to become pregnant several factors have to be normal: the man must deposit an adequate number of healthy spermatozoa in the upper part of the woman's vagina around the period of *ovulation; some sperms must be able to 'wriggle' through the twisting channels of mucus in the woman's cervix, the length of the uterus, and enter one of the Fallopian tubes; an egg (ovum) must have been discharged from the ovary and been taken into the outer portion of the Fallopian tube; one sperm must penetrate the shell of the ovum,

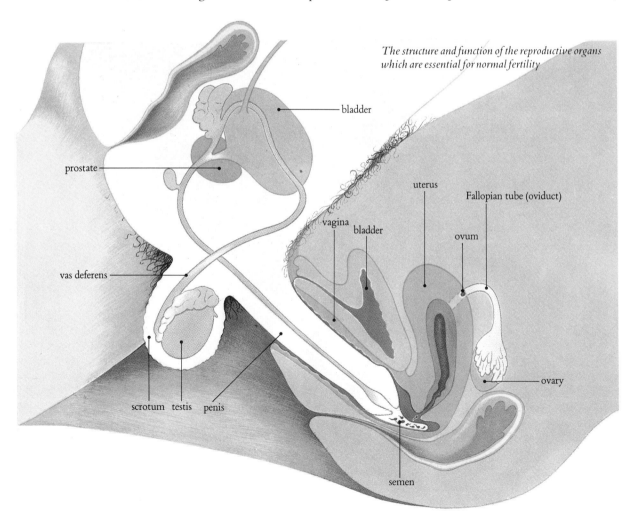

The structure and function of the reproductive organs which are essential for normal fertility

enter its cytoplasm, and fuse with its nucleus; the fertilized egg must divide several times over the following 3 to 5 days, forming a mulberry-like mass, which must enter the uterine cavity by passing along the Fallopian tube; the mulberry-like mass develops a hollow centre and is called a blastocyst. The blastocyst must be able to implant itself on the prepared lining of the uterus (endometrium) and grow into an embryo. Given the complexity of the process it is perhaps not surprising that one in every 15 couples is infertile.

Investigations usually start when the woman seeks help. At the first visit the doctor finds out about the sexual relationship of the couple, particularly the frequency of sexual intercourse. The woman also discusses her menstrual history. She is examined to make sure that she is healthy and that her genital organs are normal. The plan of the investigations is discussed. As the man is infertile in about one-third of cases, either completely or partially, it is usual for a *semen analysis to be made first to check the quantity and quality of his sperm. If this is normal, then investigations are made on the woman. Tests are made to find if she is ovulating, either by arranging for her to chart her waking temperature each day, or by measuring the level of the hormone *progesterone

in her blood. A test is then made to determine if the passage through her cervix, her uterus, and her Fallopian tubes is open or blocked. This can be carried out in two ways. In the first, called *hysterosalpingography, a substance which is opaque to X-rays is injected into the uterus and its passage through the Fallopian tubes is monitored on a television screen. The second method is to introduce an instrument called a *laparoscope into the abdomen. A laparoscope resembles a narrow telescope and enables the doctor to inspect the uterus and Fallopian tubes. A dye is injected through the cervix and the doctor watches to see if it emerges through the tubes. Other tests are sometimes carried out – for example, the *postcoital test, and biopsy of the endometrium – although many gynaecologists have found that these tests give little additional information. If it is found that *ovulation is not taking place, this may be stimulated by means of drugs (clomiphene is usually tried first). If the woman's Fallopian tubes are blocked, surgery may open them, but the success rate is less than 30 per cent (if success is defined as the birth of a healthy baby).

After all the investigations have been carried out and treatment given where necessary, between 30 and 40 per cent of infertile couples achieve a pregnancy.

Infertility, postcoital test

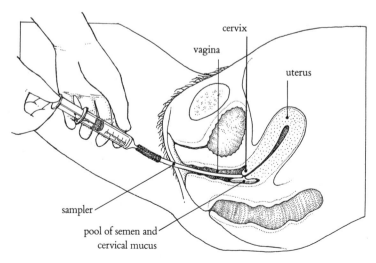

cervix

vagina

uterus

sampler

pool of semen and cervical mucus

Many gynaecologists carry out a postcoital test (Sims-Huhner test) as part of an investigation for infertility, although its usefulness has not been established. The purpose of the test is to determine firstly, if the man ejaculates spermatozoa into the vagina, and secondly, whether the secretions of the cervix are 'hostile' to the spermatozoa, preventing them from penetrating the cervical canal.

The couple have sexual intercourse at the time of *ovulation, and between 2 and 8 hours later the woman visits her doctor. He introduces a *speculum into her vagina to expose the cervix and takes a sample of the mucus secreted by the cervix and examines it under a microscope. The test is considered to be positive if 10 to 20 actively moving spermatozoa are seen. If none is observed, then either the man has failed to ejaculate in the vagina, or he has no spermatozoa in his ejaculate. A ★semen analysis is made to exclude the second possibility. If the cervical mucus contains immobile spermatozoa, cervical 'hostility' is suspected.

There are a number of problems associated with the test. Firstly, the test will be negative unless it is made between 2 days before and 1 day after ovulation, as the mucus is only receptive to spermatozoa at this time, and it is frequently difficult to detect ovulation accurately. Secondly, women who are found to have immobile spermatozoa in the cervical mucus, indicating 'hostility', have become pregnant in the same menstrual cycle. This limits the accuracy of the test.

As most women know if the man ejaculates during sexual intercourse, the first purpose of the test is limited in value. While it can be argued that the presence of semen indicates that the man is fertile, only a semen analysis can determine this accurately. The second purpose of the test is to detect cervical 'hostility', which is a possible cause of infertility in fewer than 4 per cent of couples. If *repeated* postcoital tests suggest cervical 'hostility', other tests are required to establish if an immunological antagonism exists between the spermatozoa and cervical mucus (see ★Infertility, immunological factors).

Injectable contraceptives

Although injectable contraceptives are not approved in several Western countries, they are used by nearly 2 million women in many countries. An injection of a long-acting hormone called medroxyprogesterone acetate (Depo-Provera) is given every 3 months. The hormone prevents pregnancy by suppressing ★ovulation and by changing the nature of the cervical mucus, making it 'hostile' to spermatozoa. The advantage of this form of contraception is that the hormone is taken only every 3 months. There are, however, a number of disadvantages. Firstly, the menstrual periods become disturbed: in the first 6 months, menstrual bleeding occurs at irregular, unpredictable intervals, often being scanty but annoying, and after the third injection, many women cease to menstruate. Secondly, a weight gain of 0.5 to 2.0 kg occurs over the first year. Thirdly, after the injections are stopped, periods may take up to 12 months to be re-established, and amenorrhoea can persist for over a year.

The injectables are an appropriate form of contraception for those women who choose them. As they contain no ★oestrogen, the side-effects due to that hormone are eliminated. There is no truth in the criticism that they render women permanently sterile or that they increase the risk of cancer.

Insomnia

Most people find, at some time during their life, that they are unable to sleep or that they keep waking up during the night. Sleep may be disturbed because of emotional upset, or unfamiliar surroundings, or because of pain or feelings of depression. Drugs may also cause insomnia, such as some medications or excessive amounts of coffee or tea taken in the evening. It is important to realize, however, that there is no fixed 'normal' amount of sleep. Some people need 10 hours of sleep at night, others feel and perform well on 3 hours. In general, as people grow older they need less sleep and wake more frequently during the night. Older people often 'catnap' during the day, or doze in a chair in the evening. A person's perception of how much he or she sleeps may be inaccurate, and careful studies have shown that a person may be convinced that she has not slept all night, when in fact she has had long periods of sleep. Lack of sleep is not a problem in itself and will not in itself affect a person's health – the important thing is to discover what has produced the insomnia and then to be able to correct it.

Different people have different patterns of insomnia. For example, some people find it difficult to go to sleep but once they are asleep have no problems. Other people go to sleep easily but wake up early, feeling uncomfortable. Other people wake in the middle of the night for long periods. How can you manage your insomnia? Far too many people resort to sleeping pills, which after a time become less effective, so that they have to increase the dose. Sleeping pills (or hypnotics) are useful for brief periods to restore 'normal' patterns of sleep, but if they are taken for longer periods and then stopped, a 'withdrawal' period follows which may last for up to 3 weeks, with marked insomnia. The type of hypnotic which should be taken depends on the pattern of insomnia. Barbiturates are no longer commonly prescribed and most doctors prefer to prescribe short-acting benzodiazepines (which are eliminated rapidly from the body) such as temazepam (Euhypnos, Normison), flunitrizepam (Rohypnol), or nitrazepam (Mogadon, Dormicum). A woman with insomnia should change habits which interfere with sleep.

Avoid dozing during the day.

Avoid stimulants such as tea or coffee in the late evening. Alcohol is a sedative, and may help you fall asleep but you may find that you wake up early in the morning. If you find that a glass of warm milk helps you relax, then take it.

Try to deal with any problems during the day.

Spend at least one hour before going to bed in relaxing and becoming calm.

Remember that insomnia is not a disease in itself. It is always the result of something else, and that should be treated first.

Sleeping pills taken for *short periods* help to tide you over while your doctor finds out the cause of your insomnia. But if you take them for longer periods you will find that they only help you sleep if you increase the dose, and after a while you may find it hard to give them up. If you have been taking sleeping pills for a long time, you will need help to give them up, and you must realize that you may get 'withdrawal' symptoms (particularly insomnia) which can go on for weeks.

Intrauterine device

The intrauterine device (IUD) is a small piece of plastic which has a 'memory', enabling it to return to its original shape after being stretched. In recently developed types, part of the surface of the device is covered with fine copper wire. The IUD is placed in a woman's uterus by inserting it through her cervix. In most cases it is not necessary to give an anaesthetic, but if the introduction of the IUD causes pain, the doctor should desist and introduce it on another day after giving the woman an anaesthetic. Once the IUD is placed in the uterus it usually remains there but the woman should check that the 'string' is present in her vagina after each menstrual period.

The IUD acts as a form of contraception, either by preventing spermatozoa from migrating through the uterus in search of the Fallopian tube, or by preventing the fertilized egg from implanting in the lining of the uterus (endometrium). The addition of copper wire means that a smaller device can be used, which is as effective in preventing pregnancy as the larger devices (which have no copper wire). The smaller the IUD, the fewer the side-effects. Between 5 and 15 per cent of women choose the IUD as a method of contraception. It effectively prevents pregnancy in 98 per cent of women.

The advantage of the IUD is that once the uterus has accepted it, no further contraceptive action need be taken by the woman (except for checking after each menstrual period that it has not been expelled) for 2 or 3 years. After that time the device has to be changed.

There are a number of disadvantages. First, some women develop uterine cramps and irregular bleeding in the first 2 to 4 weeks after the IUD has been inserted. The cramps can be relieved by aspirin or one of the new anti-prostaglandin drugs such as Ponstan or Naloxone. Second, menstruation tends to be heavier and to last longer. Third, if a woman becomes pregnant with an IUD in her uterus – this occurs about twice in every 100 women using an IUD for a year – *spontaneous abortion is more likely and may lead to infection. For this reason, a woman who is in this situation may wish to have the IUD removed or to have an *induced abortion. The fourth disadvantage, which is the most serious and affects about 3 women in every 1000 who have an IUD, is the occurrence of *pelvic infection or the flare-up of an existing condition. The pelvic infection may be mild, or it may be severe, in which case the Fallopian tubes may be so damaged that permanent sterility may result. Pelvic infection occurs about twice as frequently among women using an IUD as among women using other forms of contraception. If it is detected early, and treated adequately, the risk of permanent

sterility is low. For these reasons, a woman who has chosen to use an IUD should report at once to a doctor if she develops any of the following symptoms: pain and tenderness in her lower abdomen which persists for more than 24 hours; a heavy, offensive vaginal discharge; persistent pain during sexual intercourse, especially when her partner's penis thrusts deeply into her vagina. If the doctor diagnoses pelvic infection, the IUD will be removed and antibiotics prescribed.

The IUD is an excellent method of contraception for women who have side-effects from the contraceptive *pill and who find *barrier methods (condoms and diaphragms) unpleasant. It should rarely be the first contraceptive choice, however, and especially if the woman has not given birth to a baby.

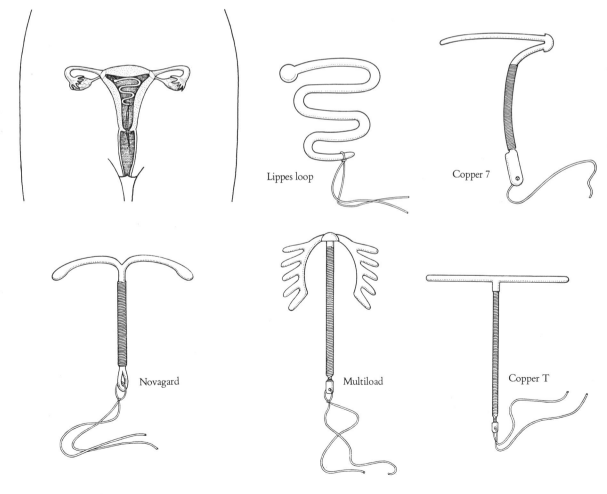

Lippes loop

Copper 7

Novagard

Multiload

Copper T

In-vitro fertilization

Women whose Fallopian tubes are irreparably damaged, or who have failed to become pregnant because of a supposed immunological barrier to spermatozoa (see *Infertility, immunological factors), may achieve a pregnancy by in-vitro fertilization of the ovum ('test-tube baby'). At an exact time just before *ovulation, the ovary which contains the ovum is visualized through a *laparoscope and the sac (follicle) containing the ovum is sucked out with a narrow needle. The fluid and the ovum are collected in a test tube. The ovum is identified and transferred to another tube containing a growth medium, and spermatozoa are added. If fertilization takes place, the fertilized egg is watched as it divides and 2 to 4 days later is gently injected into the uterus in anticipation that it will implant on the lining (endometrium) and grow. About one woman in every 10 who is treated in this way will become pregnant. All the babies born to date have been normal. As the technique requires meticulous attention to detail and is also costly, it can only be applied in a limited number of cases at the present time.

Irritable bladder

In this condition a woman has a frequent urge to pass urine, especially at night, and often experiences some discomfort when she urinates. The symptoms resemble *cystitis, but examination of the urine shows it to be sterile. The condition has an emotional origin, and various treatments have been suggested; none is entirely effective, until the underlying psychological problem is resolved. (See also *Urinary incontinence.)

Irritable bowel

This condition affects both sexes, but is more common in women. The woman complains of 'bloating' and of intermittent pain, which may be severe, in her abdomen low down on the left side. She may also complain of episodes of diarrhoea alternating with constipation. Recent research has shown that in women who have an 'irritable bowel' (or 'spastic colon') the speed with which food passes along the gut is disturbed and, in addition, the tension in the affected part of the bowel, the colon, is increased.

Irritable bowel is a psychosomatic disorder and is influenced significantly by emotional stress. Many treatments have been tried and most have failed. Currently, doctors believe the condition is helped by increasing the amount of fibre in the diet (bran is a convenient form to take) and reducing the amount of sugar, as these measures 'regularize' the movement of faeces in the gut. Drugs such as mebeverine which reduce the activity of the gut may also help. In some cases, the condition may be due to a food allergy, which can only be detected by careful dietary studies. If diarrhoea is a symptom of the irritable bowel syndrome, antiprostaglandin drugs may help prevent it.

Itching, perianal

Itchiness around the anus (the back passage) may be most distressing. In children a common cause is threadworm infestation. The female worm emerges from the anus, usually at night, to lay eggs. As she does she causes an intense irritation around the anus. The diagnosis is made by seeing the threadworms, or by taking a swabbing from the anus and sending it to a laboratory for further examination. Threadworms are most easily treated by giving a dose of a drug called Piperazine to the child and also to all other members of the family. The dose has to be repeated 14 days later.

Fungal infection of the perianal skin, usually due to *candida, is another cause of perianal itch. As with candida infection of the vagina, women who have diabetes, or who are taking antibiotics or corticosteroids are most susceptible. The diagnosis is made by taking a scraping of the skin and sending it to a laboratory. Fungal infections of the perianal skin are treated with fungicidal cream.

In a few cases of perianal itch no cause can be found, and the itch is thought to be due to psychosomatic problems.

Jaundice in the newborn

Many newborn babies are mildly jaundiced as the excess red blood cells which they required in the uterus are destroyed in the first days of life. The jaundice usually disappears within a few days. A small number of babies become more severely jaundiced soon after birth and require treatment. In some cases the baby is affected by *Rhesus iso-immune disease, in others the baby is *preterm. In these more severe cases, the paediatrician usually monitors the degree of jaundice by measuring the level of a chemical called bilirubin in a sample of the baby's blood. If the level of bilirubin exceeds a set limit, a quantity of the baby's blood is removed and is replaced by fresh blood from a donor in an exchange transfusion. In other milder cases, the baby is exposed to special light (blue light and white light) which oxidizes the bilirubin in his blood into a harmless chemical, with the result that the jaundice disappears. This treatment is known as 'phototherapy', and a baby having this will have his eyes protected by a bandage while the light is on. Sunlight is also an effective form of phototherapy.

Jaundice is more common in babies who are breast-fed, and it may be prolonged although rarely severe. It is thought to be caused by the effects of hormones in the breast milk.

K

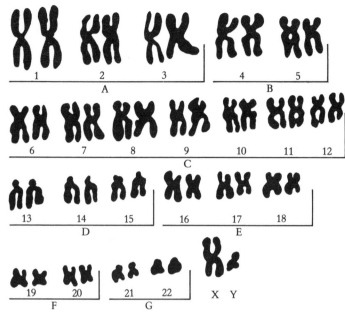

A karyotype consists of all the chromosomes of an organism. The normal karyotype of a human being has twenty-three pairs of chromosomes – the 23rd pair determines the sex

Karyotype

Just before a cell divides, its *chromosomes double in number and undergo changes which make them more obvious. It is now possible to grow human body cells in a nutrient culture and then, when they are about to divide, to add a chemical which kills the cells, fixing the chromosomes in a 'splayed-out' pattern. The cells are photographed under a microscope, and the various chromosomes are sorted into lengths and shapes which are numbered. This is called a karyotype. During pregnancy this technique is used to detect if the fetus has *Down's syndrome. An *amniocentesis is made in the 15th week of pregnancy and fetal cells, obtained from the amniotic fluid, are grown in culture and a karyotype made. In Down's syndrome, part of one of the chromosomes (no. 17) becomes detached, and resembles an extra no. 21 chromosome, so that three no. 21 chromosomes are found in the karyotype instead of the usual two.

Kegel exercises

These exercises, which were first suggested by an American physician, Dr Kegel, are designed to strengthen the muscles surrounding the vagina and rectum, for the purpose of preventing a *prolapse, reducing *urinary incontinence, and increasing sexual pleasure. The woman learns to contract and to relax the muscles which she contracts when she wants to delay or stop urinating or opening her bowels. Crudely, the exercise consists of trying to draw her back passage towards her ribcage without contracting her abdominal muscles. She contracts the muscles and counts to three, then relaxes them, and repeats the exercise between 30 and 60 times a day in batches of ten. Kegel exercises can be done anywhere: when you are sitting, walking, standing, or shopping. No one can tell if you are doing them. The effect of the exercise can be determined if the woman's partner (or doctor) places two fingers in her vagina when she does the exercise. The more tightly the fingers are gripped, the greater is the strength of the pelvic-floor muscles.

Lactation

For the mother to provide breast milk for her baby three processes have to take place. First, milk has to be secreted by the milk-producing cells in the alveoli of the breasts. Second, the milk has to be 'let down' to pass from the alveoli through the ducts to reach the reservoirs which lie deep to the nipple. Third, the baby, by suckling, has to transfer the milk from the reservoirs to his mouth. The process becomes clearer if the milk-producing parts of the breasts are visualized as a stand of between ten and twenty 'trees', the trunks of which form the main ducts which end in the nipple. The leaves of the trees are the milk-secreting sacs (alveoli), and the twigs and branches form the ductules and ducts. The 'milk trees' are embedded in fat through which blood vessels and lymphatic vessels pass like vines and creepers in a tropical forest in order to surround and supply the 'trees'.

Milk is produced by the cells of the alveoli as a result of the action of the pituitary hormone ★prolactin, which induces them to secrete milk into the hollow centre of an alveolus. The quantity of milk produced is related to the quantity of prolactin secreted, and the amount of hormone in the blood increases when the baby suckles. The more frequently he suckles, the greater the release of prolactin and the greater the quantity of milk secreted. This process is called the 'prolactin reflex'. However, the fact that milk distends the alveoli and fills the small ductules is of no benefit to the baby – it is as if the dairy has produced the milk but no trucks are available to transport it to the consumer! Milk is 'let down' from the inner part of the breast by the action of another pituitary hormone, ★oxytocin. This hormone is secreted in response to the baby suckling, although it is also released in response to psychic stimuli, such as when a mother hears her baby crying, or looks at him. When the baby suckles, messages pass to the spinal cord and from there to the brain, where they are relayed to the pituitary gland which releases oxytocin into the bloodstream. The oxytocin acts on specialized muscle cells (myoepithelial cells) which surround each group of alveolar cells. The myoepithelial cells contract and squeeze the milk out of the alveoli and eject it along the milk ducts to reach the milk reservoirs. This is called the ★milk-ejection reflex.

Laparoscope

A laparoscope is an instrument rather like a very narrow telescope which has an in-built lighting system. It is introduced into the abdomen through a small incision made just below the navel to enable the pelvic organs to be examined and abnormalities detected. The laparoscope was introduced into gynaecology about fifteen years ago and it has become very popular. Its principal place is in the diagnosis of problems connected with infertility, but it is being used increasingly to perform one method of sterilizing women in which a plastic clip kept closed by a small piece of non-corrodable sprung metal is placed across each Fallopian tube (★tubal ligation). Laparoscopy – the name given to the technique – is performed under general anaesthetic and requires an overnight stay in hospital.

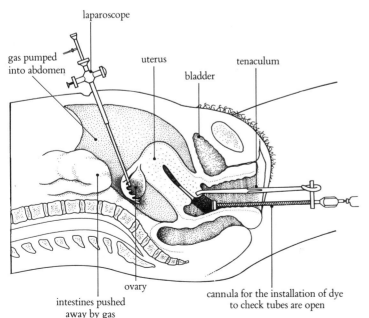

laparoscope

gas pumped into abdomen

uterus

bladder

tenaculum

intestines pushed away by gas

ovary

cannula for the installation of dye to check tubes are open

Le Boyer birth

Dr Le Boyer is a French obstetrician who has argued that the birth of a baby should be conducted in a gentle way, so that the trauma to the baby of emerging from its warm, heat-controlled, sound-proof capsule – the uterus – is minimized. Le Boyer claims that babies which are born in relative silence in a softly lit room as gently as possible adjust more easily to life outside the womb. Once born the baby is cuddled by his mother and the umbilical cord is not cut until it has ceased to pulsate. Then he is placed in a warm bath so that he can move his limbs and become accustomed to being born. The benefits of these two suggestions have not been proved, and a study comparing Le Boyer birth with a conventional but gentle and supportive approach to childbirth showed no difference in the behaviour of the mother and the baby in the first 8 months after birth. The late clamping of the cord with the baby higher than the placenta could make the baby anaemic.

The importance of Le Boyer's work lies in the fact that he reinforced the opinion that many of the methods used by health professionals during childbirth (bright lights, hard beds, clattering instruments, and so on) are not necessary. The experience of birth should be supportive and gentle and should involve both the woman and her partner in an active way.

Le Boyer's method, or one of its modifications, is now available in most Western countries, but a couple who wish to use this method of childbirth may have to look for an obstetrician who is sympathetic to Le Boyer's ideas.

Lightening

By the end of the 36th week of pregnancy, many women carrying their first baby (primigravidae) feel 'lightening'. This is because the baby's head 'drops' into the pelvic cavity; consequently, the upper part of the uterus sinks, relieving the pressure under the ribs and making breathing easier. Lightening often occurs suddenly, the woman waking up one morning relieved of the pressure and discomfort she has experienced previously. In women who have already had a child, lightening takes place later, either a week or 10 days before labour starts or in the early stages of labour.

Lochia

Lochia is the discharge which comes from the area where the *placenta was attached inside the uterus. The discharge consists of blood and the lining, or *decidua, of the uterus which is shed after childbirth. At first it is bright red and consists mainly of blood, but within a week or so its colour changes to reddish-brown, becoming yellowish-white after 3 or 4 weeks. The amount of lochia lost varies from day to day and the discharge has usually ceased within 6 weeks – the time during which orthodox Jews segregate women after childbirth, before they are allowed to have their ritual bath.

Luteal phase

After *ovulation, the follicle from which the egg (ovum) emerged collapses and forms a *corpus luteum, which secretes the sex hormone *progesterone, in addition to *oestrogen. Progesterone acts on the lining of the uterus (endometrium), making it ready to accept a fertilized egg should pregnancy occur. This phase of the menstrual cycle is called the luteal phase. In a few cases of infertility, the corpus luteum persistently fails to develop properly, with the consequence that only small quantities of progesterone are secreted, leading to a 'defective luteal phase' and perhaps sub-fertility.

Lymphogranuloma venereum

This is a sexually transmitted disease which is caused by a virus. A small lump occurs in the vulva and is followed by a rubbery enlargement of the glands in the groin, which may form abscesses. In this condition the vulva often becomes grossly swollen. Lymphogranuloma venereum is rare in developed countries, and is most common in the developing nations. The disease is treated by the use of tetracycline antibiotics.

Lymph nodes

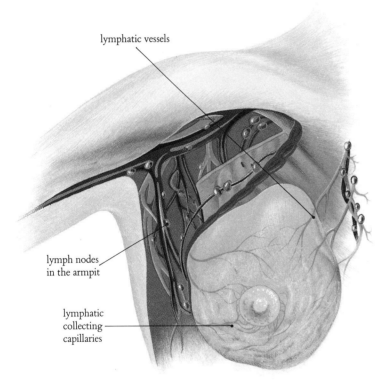

lymphatic vessels

lymph nodes in the armpit

lymphatic collecting capillaries

In addition to blood vessels, the body has a system of fine lymphatic capillaries which drain most organs and tissues. These join together to form lymphatic vessels which enter a major vein. At intervals along their course the lymphatic vessels collect into bulbous areas of lymphoid tissue, called lymph nodes. Lymph nodes 'trap' invading bacteria and become enlarged in many infections, and are important in controlling the spread of cancer as the cancer cells may be held up temporarily in the lymph nodes which drain that particular organ. For example, the lymphatic vessels of the breast drain to lymph nodes in the armpit, while those from the uterus drain into lymph nodes on the inner wall of the pelvis. In surgery for *breast cancer, it is usual to remove as many of the lymph nodes in the armpit as possible so that they may be checked for the presence or absence of cancer cells. If the lymph nodes contain no cancer cells, the woman's chances of survival are much higher than if they are involved. In this case, additional treatment such as radiotherapy or *chemotherapy may be suggested.

M

Mammography

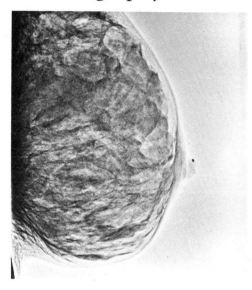

A mammogram of a normal breast

Mammography is a technique of examining a woman's breasts using X-rays. The use of special films means that only a very small dose of radiation is absorbed by the woman's tissues, which makes the procedure relatively safe. Mammography is valuable because it enables doctors to detect *breast lumps which may be cancerous at a very early stage, usually earlier than they can be detected by clinical examination of the breast. The earlier breast cancer is detected, the greater is the chance of cure. However, some radiation is absorbed by the woman during mammography, and this may induce cancer if the examination is repeated often. It has been calculated that if 1 million women were examined each year from the age of 30, about 230 excess breast cancers might develop. Against this, mammography would *save* at least that many women by detecting breast cancer early.

The present advice is that mammography is an appropriate investigation for all women aged 40 and more, and for younger women who are at higher risk of developing breast cancer because a close relative has developed the disease. If women are examined by mammography, an abnormal appearance in the X-ray film will lead to the recommendation for further examination by a doctor in 5 per cent of women and for a breast biopsy (where a small piece of tissue is removed for examination) in one or two women in every 100. Of the women who undergo a breast biopsy only one in 5 will have breast cancer.

Manchester operation

This is an operation for *prolapse, so called because the technique was devised about eighty years ago by two surgeons from Manchester. Prolapse was relatively common in the North of England and was believed to be due to frequent childbearing, poor care during childbirth, and the resumption of heavy work too soon after childbirth. In prolapse, the uterus 'falls' and the cervix becomes elongated, and the vaginal walls stretch as its muscle is weakened. The Manchester operation shortened the cervix, narrowed the vagina, and strengthened its supporting muscles. The technique is still used, but often a vaginal *hysterectomy is performed instead of shortening the cervix.

Mastectomy

Each year between 2 and 4 women in every 1000 aged 40 or over are found to have *breast cancer. Treatment is to remove the affected breast surgically, but the more radical operations of past years have now largely been abandoned. However, the loss of a breast by mastectomy causes considerable psychological stress. Breasts have a strong erotic connotation and are symbolic of femininity and womanhood. The loss of a breast

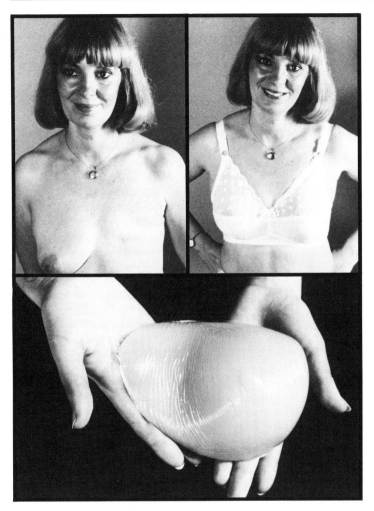

implies a reduction in femininity and the fear that the woman will be less desirable sexually and socially; this occurs at a time when she is also trying to come to terms with the knowledge that she has cancer. The loss of her body-image may diminish the woman's self-esteem and she may become depressed for several months, or withdraw from her relationships. To minimize this loss, women who have had a mastectomy have come together to form voluntary helping organizations. These women visit the patient both while she is in hospital and later at home, if she requests it, to give advice and support. It is usual for the woman to receive a temporary breast shape (prosthesis) while still in hospital, which can be worn in a bra so that she looks normal when she leaves. Later, when the scar is no longer tender, she can buy a permanent prosthesis of the right size and shape (see opposite).

New techniques are now available in which the surgeon reconstructs the breast, some six months after mastectomy, by inserting a silicone breast prosthesis under the skin and making a new nipple. The operation is relatively simple and the stay in hospital need not be longer than one or two days. A breast reconstruction gives the woman the additional psychological benefit that she no longer has to wear a prosthesis to look 'normal' and no longer has to confront the fact that she has only one breast when she changes her clothes, bathes, or goes to bed.

Masturbation

Most males and females obtain sexual pleasure by touching and stroking their external genital organs. This is called masturbation. A male plays with and strokes his penis to obtain sexual pleasure; a female plays with or strokes the area around her clitoris. During masturbation, most people have sexual fantasies, and reach orgasm, which may be equally or more intense than orgasm obtained during *sexual intercourse or *oral sex. Masturbation is a normal sexual outlet; it causes no physical or mental damage to most people but it may arouse feelings of guilt in a few. It does not lead to impotence,

heavy menstrual periods, blindness, mental decay, or premature senility – consequences which until recently were said to result from masturbation.

Masturbation has several benefits. During sexual development it enables the person to learn his or her response to sexual stimulation. It teaches women to explore and to understand their genital anatomy. When a person is separated from a lover by distance or by death, masturbation provides a way of obtaining sexual relief without the need to find a new partner. Masturbation is a personal matter, and one of individual choice.

Maternal mortality

It has been agreed internationally that maternal death shall be defined as 'the death of any woman dying from any cause whilst pregnant or within 42 days of the termination of pregnancy, irrespective of the duration and the size of the pregnancy, from any cause related to or aggravated by pregnancy and its management'. Most countries which accept the definition report the deaths as a rate per 100000 'maternities', which includes all pregnancies ending with livebirth or stillbirth. Some countries (for example, the United Kingdom) extend the period after the termination of pregnancy to 1 year.

Between 1880 and 1934, the death rate of pregnant and puerperal (lying-in) women in the United Kingdom and other developed countries fluctuated, remaining stubbornly between 500 and 700 per 100000 births (between 5 and 7 per cent). Since 1934, a remarkable change has occurred: the maternal mortality rate has fallen to between 6 and 12 per 100000 maternities.

The improvement has been due to a number of factors: better nutrition in childhood and adolescence; the general availability and acceptance of *antenatal care; the decision made by women to have fewer children, at an earlier age; the provision of specialist training in obstetrics for doctors and nurses; the provision of well-equipped maternity hospitals, with good facilities for anaesthesia, blood transfusion, and monitoring.

This means that today pregnancy and childbirth have become safe for women, provided that they avail themselves of the facilities that are provided.

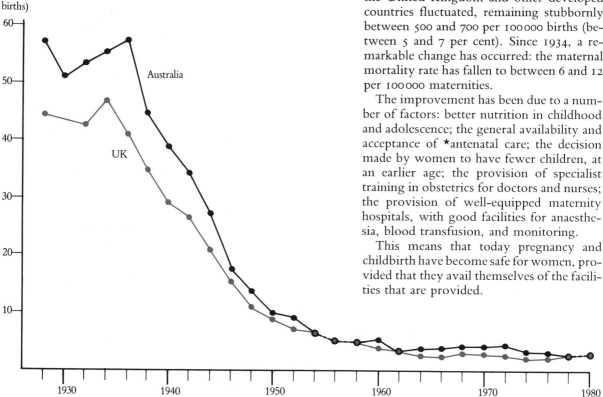

Maternal deaths (per 10,000 live births)

Menarche

The menarche means the start of menstrual periods, which is a significant event in the life of a woman. Menarche usually occurs at about the age of 12½, but it is quite normal for menstruation to start as early as the age of 9 or as late as 17.

The reason why a girl starts to menstruate is still unclear, but a considerable amount has been learned in the past ten years. There seems to be a critical body weight-for-height which a girl has to achieve before menstruation starts. If the girl is thin, and particularly if she exercises very hard so that she has little body fat – for example, if she is at a ballet-school or takes part in competitive swimming – her menarche may be delayed.

How this important weight-for-height ratio is involved in the onset of menstruation is unknown, because the essential change which triggers menstruation takes place in the brain. In childhood, a brain hormone called gonadotrophic releasing hormone (GnRH) is released steadily and at a low level. In the years before the menarche, a change occurs and GnRH is released in pulses. These pulsed surges of GnRH stimulate the release of hormones from the pituitary gland and these in turn stimulate the ovaries to make and to release *oestrogen. Oestrogen stimulates the uterus to grow and eventually to bleed: the first menstrual period. In many cultures this marks the girl's transition from childhood to womanhood when she is capable of bearing children. In Western society, although the onset of womanhood is considered important, menstruation often cannot be talked about openly. Usually the girl's mother talks with her, and other information is obtained from school, books, or talking with her friends, but some girls lack accurate knowledge. Most girls perceive menarche as an emotional event, and many describe themselves as being scared, upset, angry, or tearful.

Menopause

Menopause means the cessation of menstruation, the main event marking a woman's transition from the years when reproduction is possible to the post-reproductive .years. This period of transition is associated with hormonal changes in the woman's body and more correct terms to describe it are the 'climateric' or the 'change of life'. However, 'menopause' is now used interchangeably with climacteric to describe this time in a woman's life.

The hormonal changes begin early in the fifth decade of a woman's life, when the level of one of the pituitary hormones (gonadotrophins) which stimulate the ovaries increases in relation to the other. The altered ratio between the hormones disturbs the function of the ovaries, resulting in less frequent *ovulation and often in an alteration in menstruation, which may become irregular in duration or in frequency. As the years pass, the responsiveness of the ovaries to the gonadotrophins diminishes further, less *oestrogen is secreted, and finally menstruation ceases at about the age of 51. Menopause has occurred.

Although the hormonal changes are the cause of some of the menopausal symptoms, psychosocial factors are also involved. In a youth-oriented society, a woman reaching menopause may note that she is seen as middle-aged (and may consequently feel middle-aged) and that she is no longer capable of childbearing. Her children have either left home or are no longer dependent on her or deferential to her. Her relationship with her husband (or partner) may have deteriorated. If she reaches menopause at this stage in her life, she may blame her depression, anxiety, fatigue, and irritability on her hormones rather than on the psychosocial upset.

The main hormonal changes which occur in the years around menopause and which produce symptoms are a rapid decline in the level of oestrogen and an increase in the level of gonadotrophins circulating in the woman's body. Oestrogen deficiency is the cause of the *hot flushes (with associated insomnia and sweating) which may make a woman's life a misery. It is also a factor in the vaginal dryness which may occur at menopause, but usually occurs later, and which makes *sexual intercourse uncomfortable. Oestrogen deficiency (together with a lack of exercise and a lack of calcium absorbed by the intestines) is involved in *osteoporosis which affects many women in their sixties or seventies.

These particular symptoms of oestrogen deficiency can be relieved by *hormone replacement therapy. However, the many other symptoms which are reported by menopausal women are not due to lack of oestrogen, and hormone replacement therapy is not indicated. As *unopposed* oestrogen therapy is associated with an increase in *endometrial cancer, and perhaps in coronary heart disease and breast cancer, the following guidelines for oestrogen therapy should be observed: the oestrogen should be taken in the smallest effective dose which relieves the symptoms and should be taken for the shortest period of time; *gestagen should be given for about 12 days each month together with oestrogen; the dose must be adjusted so that it is appropriate for each woman. Oestrogen prescribed in this way has proved a boon to women suffering from menopausal symptoms due to oestrogen deficiency, and is safe. The hormone is now made in the laboratory and several formulations are available, none of which is demonstrably superior to any of the others. Oestrogen is normally taken by mouth, but is available as a pessary or a cream which is inserted in the vagina where it is readily absorbed.

As many problems which occur in the years around the menopause may be due to the woman's altered perception of her worth to her husband, to her children, and to society, discussion about these matters may prove helpful, either with a sympathetic friend or relative, or if the problems are severe with a trained counsellor.

Menstrual hygiene

Until seventy years ago, women used pieces of cloth to soak up the flow of blood during menstruation. These 'rags' were washed and used again. Today commercial manufacturers produce a variety of products for menstrual hygiene. *Sanitary pads* (or towels) which are worn with a belt have been used for several decades. *Beltless sanitary pads* are also available; they have a strip of adhesive on the underside so that they can be attached to panties or pantihose. External sanitary pads should be changed about every 4 hours to prevent unpleasant odour. Many women prefer to use *tampons*; these are inserted into the vagina, either with the fingers or by means of the cardboard or plastic applicator which is withdrawn when the tampon is in place. Tampons should not be used continually throughout a menstrual period, as this may lead (rarely) to *toxic shock. They should be changed every 4 hours during the day, and an external sanitary pad worn at night.

Most young women choose sanitary pads when they first start menstruating, but by the age of 17 increasing numbers use tampons, particularly if they are sexually active. Manufacturers have produced very slim tampons which can be used by women who have not had *sexual intercourse; and thicker, more absorbent tampons for women who have heavy periods.

It used to be commonly believed that a woman should not bathe or wash her hair during a menstrual period, but this is untrue. There is no reason why normal hygienic habits should not be continued, and daily washing or bathing is in fact important during menstruation, both for cleanliness and to make a woman feel fresh and comfortable.

Menstrual problems

The main menstrual problems are painful periods (*dysmenorrhoea) and menstrual irregularities. The menstrual periods usually occur at intervals of 24 to 35 days, counting day 1 as the day bleeding starts, and last for between 2 and 7 days. The amount of blood lost ranges from 10 to 80 mls (averaging 35 mls) and bleeding is considered heavy if more than 80 mls is lost. Menstruation may occur at intervals shorter than 21 days, or longer than 35 days, and this may cause anxiety or be inconvenient. If this happens, a doctor should be consulted. The amount of blood lost may be scanty (which is usually not a cause of worry) or heavy, when discomfort or pain caused by clots being expelled from the uterus may occur and when iron-deficiency *anaemia may result. This condition of unusually heavy periods, called menorrhagia, requires further investigation. Menorrhagia may be due to *fibroids, or may be associated with *pelvic infection, but often it is due to an imbalance in the production of pituitary and ovarian hormones. The investigations will establish the cause. If no uterine disease is found, the condition is called dysfunctional uterine bleeding. Treatment of this condition depends on the age of the woman, her desire to retain her child-bearing potential, and the severity of the bleeding. Usually, a *D and C is carried out, or hormone treatment (using *gestagens) is prescribed. In some more extreme cases a *hysterectomy may be the suggested treatment.

Some women develop irregular bleeding, when the interval may range from one or two days to 3 weeks or more and the amount of blood lost vary from scanty to heavy. This should be investigated by a doctor as the bleeding may be caused by a tumour of the uterus or *ovaries, although in many cases it is due to a hormonal disturbance, as are the other menstrual irregularities. Absence or the stopping of periods during the reproductive years of a woman is most commonly due to pregnancy, but occasionally *amenorrhoea occurs; this condition should be investigated if the periods do not recommence in 6 to 9 months.

Menstrual regulation

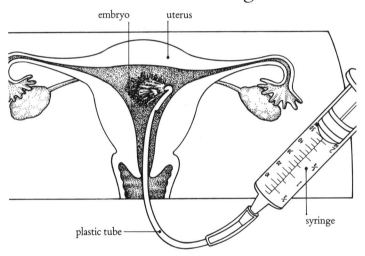

Menstrual regulation, emptying the uterus by means of suction if menstruation does not occur, has been introduced as a means of controlling pregnancy. Most pregnancy tests do not become positive until the 40th day after the last menstrual period, and before this time pregnancy is only suspected. If a woman thinks it is possible that she has become pregnant and her menstrual period is 7 days overdue, she visits a doctor for 'menstrual regulation'. He inserts a narrow plastic tube into her uterus, attaches it to a large syringe, and empties the uterus. If the woman is pregnant, the embryo (which is only 5 mm long) is sucked out with the lining of the uterus (endometrium); if she is not pregnant, only endometrium is removed. No anaesthesia is required. The choice of menstrual regulation as a method of pregnancy control avoids the moral question of knowing that the woman was pregnant. Sometimes the embryo is not sucked out of the uterus and the pregnancy continues.

Menstruation, attitudes towards

In most societies, including Western society until recently, menstruation was considered a secretive, rather shameful matter. Even today with a wider dissemination of knowledge about menstruation, teenagers tend to perceive menstruation in a negative manner, as a time of discomfort or inconvenience which interferes with school-work and sport. These attitudes towards menstruation may derive from messages given by the girl's mother or her friends who may refer to menstruation as 'the poorly time' or 'the curse'; or they may derive from books or pamphlets the girl has read. Too often, published sources take menarche and menstruation out of context and imply that this is a time of mystery, embarrassment, and privacy. They tend to emphasize how the girl should feel and what she should do for *menstrual hygiene, rather than allowing the girl to make her own assessment of her feelings towards menstruation.

The girl's cultural background also affects her attitude towards menstruation. Certain ethnic groups see the main reason for menstruation as a method whereby the body rids itself of impurities. They believe that unless the blood flows freely, the impurities will not be discharged, so that it is essential to avoid cold and certain medications. Menstruation is also seen as weakening, so the woman must not exert herself and should be careful as infection can 'get into' her body, especially through her genital tract during menstruation.

These negative feelings towards menstruation are not confined to lower classes or particular ethnic communities. In a study of college students in the United States in 1980, certain common attitudes to menstruation emerged. These were that menstruation is natural but bothersome, and not debilitating.

However, it should be kept secret and the girl should 'act normally and not let menstruation affect you'. Many teenage girls are affected by strange attitudes to menstruation and believe that during menstruation they should avoid exercise, swimming, going out in the cold, and washing their hair. This is a legacy of the erroneous theories of doctors in the nineteenth century who believed that exposure to cold during menstruation caused inflammation of the lining of the uterus. 'Such an inflammation once excited will often go on for years and in time end in dysmenorrhoea, sterility, pelvic pain, and gastric disorders, which impair digestion and nutrition', one doctor wrote in 1880. Menstruation has no damaging effect on the body, and during menstruation a woman can undertake any activity, including sexual intercourse, that she wishes.

Menstruation, normal

Menstruation is the end of a complicated series of hormonal interactions which occur in a woman's body each month. It is easier to understand the process by starting at the end of menstruation. At this time the level of *oestrogen circulating in the blood is relatively low. This permits the pituitary gland to secrete a hormone called follicle stimulating hormone (FSH) which circulates in the blood and is taken up by the tissues of the ovaries where it stimulates between 10 and 20 of the tiny egg nests, or *egg follicles, to grow. The follicles increase in size, one growing faster than the others, and as they grow they secrete oestrogen into the blood. The rising levels of oestrogen 'feed back' to the part of the brain called the hypothalamus; from there a message is sent to the pituitary gland and the amount of FSH which is released into the blood decreases. The level of oestrogen in the blood continues to rise and reaches a peak. This causes a sudden surge of a hormone to be released in the hypothalamus which is carried by a system of blood vessels to the pituitary gland. There it stimulates the release of a surge of FSH, and a much larger surge of a second hormone, luteinizing hormone (LH). LH is carried in

the blood to the ovary where it is absorbed into the largest follicle, which by now is stretching the surface of the ovary. LH induces the follicle to burst, releasing the egg (ovum) which is taken into the Fallopian tube. This is called *ovulation. When the egg has been expelled, the follicle collapses. Its cells turn yellow, to form a *corpus luteum (yellow body) which secretes the second ovarian hormone *progesterone as well as oestrogen.

Under the influence of the rising levels of oestrogen, the lining of the uterus (endometrium) has been growing thicker. Its glands become longer, and the cells between them become larger. Progesterone now induces the glands to produce mucus, they become twisted, and the cells between them become larger still. The endometrium is being prepared for a possible pregnancy. If the egg is fertilized, it starts dividing and 5 days after ovulation reaches the cavity of the uterus and implants into the endometrium. If the egg is not fertilized, the corpus luteum ages and dies about 12 to 14 days after ovulation. Consequently, the levels of oestrogen and progesterone fall. This causes the blood vessels which supply the endometrium to kink, so

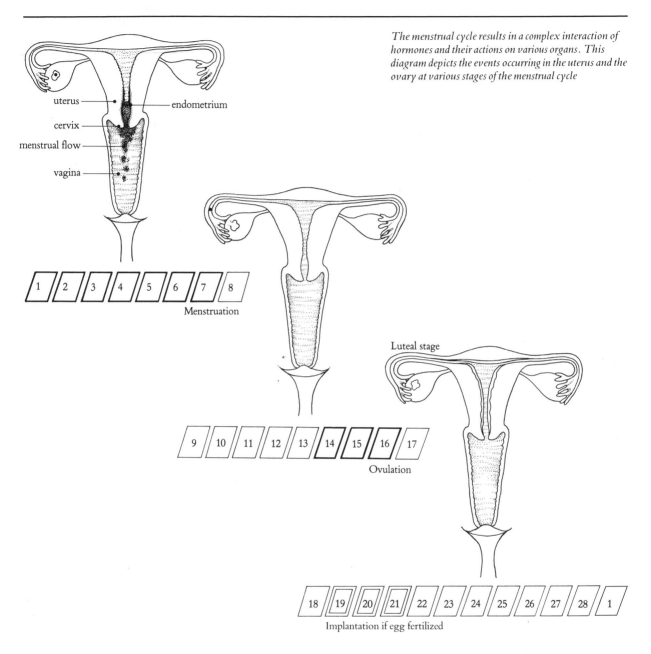

The menstrual cycle results in a complex interaction of hormones and their actions on various organs. This diagram depicts the events occurring in the uterus and the ovary at various stages of the menstrual cycle

uterus — endometrium

cervix

menstrual flow

vagina

| 1 | 2 | 3 | 4 | 5 | 6 | 7 | 8 |

Menstruation

| 9 | 10 | 11 | 12 | 13 | 14 | 15 | 16 | 17 |

Ovulation

Luteal stage

| 18 | 19 | 20 | 21 | 22 | 23 | 24 | 25 | 26 | 27 | 28 | 1 |

Implantation if egg fertilized

that less blood runs through them. Deprived of blood, the surface layers of the endometrium die in patches, and blood seeps from the damaged vessels. The blood and the surface layers of the endometrium collect in the cavity of the uterus. The blood clots dissolve, and the liquid blood emerges through the cervix. Menstruation has begun. By now the level of FSH is beginning to rise and to stimulate a new group of follicles to repeat the menstrual cycle.

Menstruation usually lasts for between 2 and 7 days and between 10 and 80 mls (averaging 35 mls) of blood are lost. The menstrual cycle, which is counted from the first day of bleeding (day 1) to the last day before the next menstrual period, lasts between 24 and 35 days in 95 per cent of women.

Mental handicap and sexuality
Metabolic diseases of the newborn
Milk-ejection reflex

Mental handicap and sexuality

With improved health care, increasing numbers of mentally handicapped children, especially those with ★Down's syndrome, reach adolescence and adulthood. About 2 per cent of the population are mentally retarded and until recently society repressed the expression of their sexuality by segregating them. However, 9 out of 10 of those who are mentally retarded are capable of functioning in a sheltered environment and may wish to form sexual relationships.

Parents' feelings about the sexuality of their mentally retarded child range from the belief that it is better to keep the young woman 'innocent' through over-protection, as sex is regarded as too 'risky', to a moralistic view that sex is sinful for a retarded person. These opinions conflict with the reality: mentally retarded people do have sexual feelings, which are usually expressed initially by ★masturbation. Parents should not try to prevent their retarded child from actively masturbating, as it is pleasurable, but they should ensure by firm training that the child only masturbates in appropriate places. The second main concern of parents is that their mentally retarded child will be exploited sexually. The chance of sexual exploitation can be minimized if the parents teach the child specific behaviours rather than keeping him or her under constant observation. There is evidence that sex education given by trained counsellors helps a retarded adolescent girl to understand and interpret her sexual urges and to cope more successfully with them than if she is kept ignorant. If two retarded people form a relationship, the chance that it will become a sexual relationship should be anticipated, not by separating the couple, but by ensuring that contraception is provided. Such relationships are usually beneficial to the couple, providing affection, preventing loneliness, and enabling them to live a life as normal as possible.

Metabolic diseases of the newborn

Three congenital (inborn) metabolic defects which can cause serious illness in a baby unless treated can be detected in the first days after birth. These are *phenylketonuria* (one in every 10000 births), *congenital hypothyroidism* (one in every 6000 births), and *cystic fibrosis* (one in every 2000 births). Unless phenylketonuria is detected soon after birth, a baby with this enzyme defect accumulates a substance called phenylalanine which comes from protein in his food. Over a number of months, the accumulation of phenylalanine causes irreversible mental retardation. This can be prevented if the baby is given a diet which is low in phenylalanine content. A baby suffering from congenital hypothyroidism has insufficient thyroid hormone in his blood and will become intellectually handicapped and a cretin unless treated. Cystic fibrosis is a disease which causes repeated chest infections and lung damage, together with malnutrition. Early diagnosis and special treatment will help to prevent lung damage from becoming serious.

The three diseases can be diagnosed by taking a drop of blood from the baby's heel on the fifth day after birth. The blood is put on special filter paper which is sent to a laboratory for testing. The test is sometimes called the Guthrie test.

Milk-ejection reflex

After childbirth, milk is produced in the small sacs (alveoli) which lie deep in the tissues of the breast; these correspond to the leaves of the 'milk tree' (see ★Breast anatomy). Milk secretion is stimulated by suckling, and this also initiates the milk-ejection ('let-down') reflex. The production of milk depends on the interplay of a number of hormones, of which ★prolactin is the principal one. However, none of these hormones

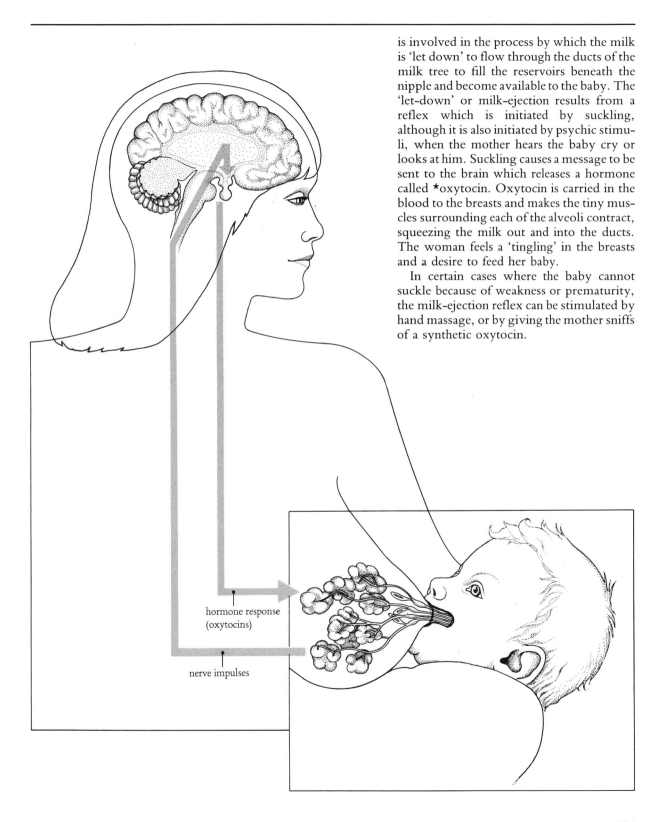

hormone response
(oxytocins)

nerve impulses

is involved in the process by which the milk is 'let down' to flow through the ducts of the milk tree to fill the reservoirs beneath the nipple and become available to the baby. The 'let-down' or milk-ejection results from a reflex which is initiated by suckling, although it is also initiated by psychic stimuli, when the mother hears the baby cry or looks at him. Suckling causes a message to be sent to the brain which releases a hormone called ★oxytocin. Oxytocin is carried in the blood to the breasts and makes the tiny muscles surrounding each of the alveoli contract, squeezing the milk out and into the ducts. The woman feels a 'tingling' in the breasts and a desire to feed her baby.

In certain cases where the baby cannot suckle because of weakness or prematurity, the milk-ejection reflex can be stimulated by hand massage, or by giving the mother sniffs of a synthetic oxytocin.

Mini-pill

The so-called Mini-pill (progestogen-only pill) is a hormone contraceptive pill which contains no *oestrogen, relying for its effect on the second hormone, *gestagen (progestogen). The Mini-pill has to be taken every day, whether there is bleeding or not, and it is best taken in the evening. The Mini-pill prevents pregnancy in two ways. First, it alters the character of the cervical mucus so that the sperms find it more difficult to wriggle through. Second, it also probably alters the lining of the woman's uterus (endometrium) so that it becomes less suitable for implantation by an egg should one be fertilized by chance.

The Mini-pill is not as efficient in protecting a woman against becoming pregnant as the combined *pill, and between 2 and 4 in every 100 women using it will become pregnant each year. It should therefore only be chosen if the woman cannot take a pill containing oestrogen (because of the side-effects it causes) or if she is breast-feeding (since a pill containing oestrogen may reduce the quantity of milk).

The side-effects of the Mini-pill are annoying rather than dangerous. Menstrual periods tend to be unpredictable both in the amount of blood lost and in the time of onset; they may be more frequent, occurring at longer intervals, they may become very irregular, or frequent small blood losses may occur daily. After a woman has taken the Mini-pill for a few months, the absence of periods (the condition known as *amenorrhoea) becomes increasingly common.

Mittelschmerz

A proportion of women complain during their reproductive years of lower abdominal pain or discomfort which occurs about halfway between their menstrual periods. The pain is felt on one or other side of the abdomen, and usually it will only last a few hours.

Typically the abdominal pain recurs most months, but occasionally it may be absent. This pain, which is called mittelschmerz, is due to *ovulation, and occurs when the follicle which contains the egg stretches the surface of the ovary and subsequently bursts, thus releasing the egg.

Morning-after pill

A single act of unprotected sexual intercourse at the time of *ovulation, halfway between menstrual periods, is statistically likely to be followed by a pregnancy in 20 to 30 per cent of women aged 15 to 45. The woman has two choices. The first is to wait to see if menstruation occurs, and if it does not then either to continue the pregnancy or to seek an abortion. The second choice is to use the 'morning-after' pill ('postcoital contraception'), which is a high-dose contraceptive pill (for example, Ovral or Eugynon). Two pills are taken, followed by another two 12 hours later. In order to be effective in preventing pregnancy, the first dose must be taken within 72 hours of the man's ejaculation in the woman's vagina. The drug is associated with nausea (sometimes vomiting) and should be used for emergencies only, such as following *rape or a single act of intercourse. It is not suitable for routine use over the 7 days in the middle of the menstrual cycle as it would have to be taken too frequently and the total dose of hormones which it contains is higher than that in a low-dose pill.

There is also some concern that the hormones contained in the morning-after pill may cause damage to the embryo if the pregnancy occurs in spite of taking the pill. The evidence is that this is unlikely, but a woman may choose to have an abortion should the morning-after pill fail to cause the onset of menstruation.

Mother love

The traditional view is that a mother loves her baby the moment he is born. This view is alarming, as experience shows that some mothers do not have this instinctive love for the baby, and may feel that there is something wrong with them. One study carried out in New South Wales, Australia, found that only 59 per cent of women felt 'mother love' in the first week of the baby's life; by the end of the third week the percentage had risen to 82 per cent, and by the 12th week nearly all the women felt love for their baby. This would seem to indicate that mother love may take time to develop.

Multiple pregnancy

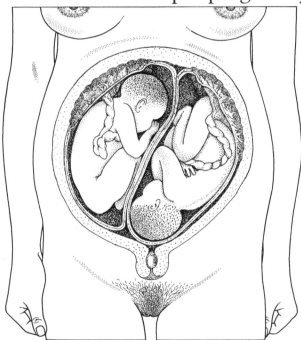

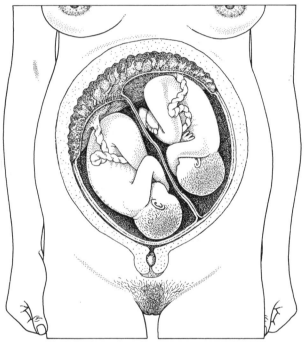

Fraternal twins produced by the chance fertilization of two ova

Identical twins, produced from the fertilization of one ova which divides into two identical embryos

Multiple pregnancy occurs when two (or more) eggs are released from the ovary and are fertilized simultaneously, or when a single fertilized egg divides into two separate eggs.

Twins occur once in every 90 pregnancies, triplets once in every 90 × 90 pregnancies, and quadruplets once in every 90 × 90 × 90 pregnancies. As twins are the most common form of multiple pregnancy, they will be considered in detail. If two eggs are released and fertilized simultaneously, the twins are fraternal: that is, they are no more close to each other in genetic make-up than are other brothers or sisters. If a single egg is fertilized and divides equally to form two separate individuals, the twins are identical in genetic make-up (uniovular twins).

Twins may be diagnosed by *ultrasound in early pregnancy, by ultrasound or X-ray in mid-pregnancy, and clinically in late pregnancy. A woman carrying twins has a more enlarged abdomen and more chance of developing *pre-eclampsia and iron-deficiency *anaemia than a mother carrying one baby. Perhaps the most serious problems of twins are that at every stage of pregnancy each baby tends to be smaller than a singleton baby at the same stage, and *premature (preterm) labour is more common, between one-quarter and one-third of babies of multiple pregnancies being born before the 36th week. If the woman takes increased rest in the last 10 weeks of pregnancy the chance of preterm birth is said to be reduced, but this has recently been disputed. Because of the increased weight she is carrying, the woman may be more tired and may require more rest. In addition, she needs to take iron and folic acid tablets because the two babies put increased demands on her.

Childbirth takes no longer than for singleton births. Once the first twin has been born, the doctor usually examines the woman vaginally and breaks the bag of waters surrounding the second twin so that it is born quickly.

Twins require more attention than singleton births, and in some countries Multiple Birth Associations exist which offer support and advice to parents. Mothers find it easier to breast-feed twins than to prepare bottles and feed them with formula milk foods. Most mothers who give birth to twins ultimately seem to find the experience very rewarding.

Myths about women

It is perhaps surprising that despite a much wider dissemination of sexual information nowadays, especially through the media, and less reticence about talking and reading about sexual matters, many women, and more men, believe in myths which derive from ignorance and folklore. Some of these myths are listed here.

Anatomy
Some women can trap a man's penis in the vagina.
Some women can't have sex because their vagina is too small or the man's penis is too large.

Breasts
Women are unconcerned about the size of their breasts.
Large breasts indicate the woman is likely to be more interested in sex.
Women with small breasts are unable to breast-feed successfully.
Breast-feeding leads to sagging breasts.
Hair on the area around the nipples indicates that the woman is abnormal.
All women enjoy having their breasts fondled.
Women with big breasts are very fertile.

Contraception
Douching is an effective method of contraception.
Passing urine after intercourse prevents pregnancy.
After tubal ligation a woman becomes fat and loses interest in sex.
Sterilization means the ovaries are removed.
A man who has had a vasectomy does not ejaculate.
The pill leads to promiscuity.
The pill leads to sterility.

Homosexuality
Lesbians are all 'butch'.
Lesbians cannot form lasting relationships.
Women who enjoy sports are likely to be lesbian.

Masturbation
Women do not masturbate.
Masturbation is a sign that a woman cannot form a good relationship.
Excessive masturbation causes weakness and physical illness.
Women who need a vibrator are oversexed.
Married women do not masturbate.
In pregnancy, masturbation can cause an abortion or bring on labour.
Masturbation may make a woman sterile.

Menstruation
Women cannot be trusted in important positions because they become irrational in the week before and during menstruation.
Menstruation cleans the body of dirty blood.
A woman should douche when menstruation finishes.
Intercourse should be avoided during menstruation as the man's penis may introduce infection or damage her fragile tissues, and the menstrual blood may damage his penis.
Menstruation is weakening, so a woman should not play active sports during a period.

A woman should not get cold or wash her hair during menstruation as the blood may not flow out easily and this may lead to disease.

Oral sex

Oral sex is unnatural.

Women who swallow semen will do themselves damage.

If a pregnant woman swallows semen she will abort or labour will be started.

Rape (sexual assault)

Rapists are usually strangers.

Rapists are sexually unfulfilled men who have sudden uncontrollable urges.

Rapists are mentally ill and not responsible for their behaviour.

Women are raped because they ask for it by wearing seductive clothes and behaving provocatively.

A woman cannot be raped unless she wants to be.

A woman who hitch-hikes or goes alone to pubs is asking to be raped.

Most women really want to be raped.

Sex-roles

Women who have careers make poor mothers.

Unless a woman marries and has children she has failed to fulfil her biological destiny.

Sex is not very important to a woman except as a means of making her man happy.

A woman should not compete with, or surpass, her man.

Women who make the first move towards a man are promiscuous.

Sexual intercourse

The only proper way to have intercourse is with the man on top.

If the woman is on top, it shows that the man is weak and the woman is a nymphomaniac.

A woman cannot become pregnant if she has intercourse standing up.

Sensitive lovers use many different positions for intercourse.

Pregnant women lose all interest in sex.

In the first quarter of pregnancy, sexual intercourse will cause an abortion.

In the last weeks of pregnancy, sexual intercourse will bring on labour prematurely and may harm the baby.

If the man has sexual intercourse lying on top of his pregnant partner he will damage the baby.

If a woman does not have an orgasm she will not get pregnant.

As women grow older they lose their desire for sex.

A woman who does not have an orgasm simultaneously with the man is frigid.

A man can tell if a woman will be good in bed by the shape of her hips.

N

Nabothian cyst

These are small cysts which are found under the surface of the *cervix. They are caused when a new growth of surface cells covers and blocks the outlet of one of the glands in the cervix which secrete a thick mucus. If the outlet becomes blocked, the mucus collects and distends the gland, forming a small cyst. Nabothian cysts are harmless and can be left untreated, or the doctor may puncture the cyst with a hot cautery needle.

Natural family planning: the mucus method

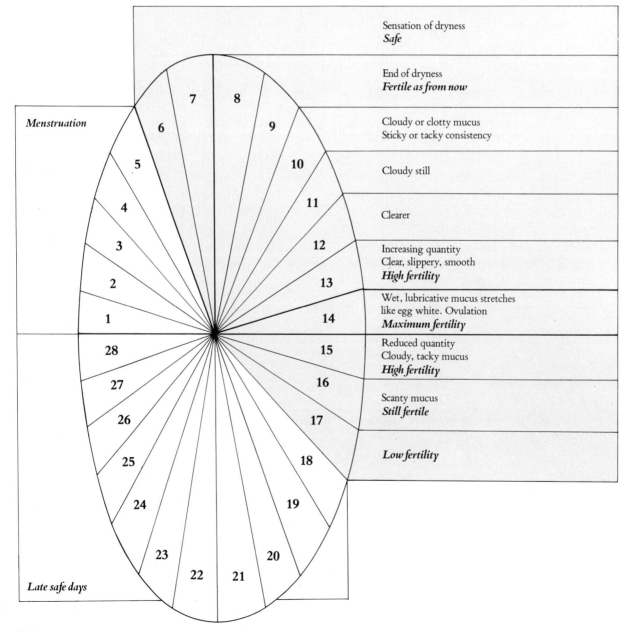

Menstruation

Late safe days

Sensation of dryness
Safe

End of dryness
Fertile as from now

Cloudy or clotty mucus
Sticky or tacky consistency

Cloudy still

Clearer

Increasing quantity
Clear, slippery, smooth
High fertility

Wet, lubricative mucus stretches like egg white. Ovulation
Maximum fertility

Reduced quantity
Cloudy, tacky mucus
High fertility

Scanty mucus
Still fertile

Low fertility

Natural family planning: the mucus method
the sympto-thermal method
the calendar method

This method of avoiding pregnancy by 'natural' means depends on the known fact that in the 4 or 5 days before and the 3 to 4 days after *ovulation, the cervix of the uterus secretes a clear, stretchy mucus in considerable quantity. In the days after menstruation, the cervical mucus is scanty and thick and, in general, none is found at the vaginal entrance, which is now dry. As ovulation approaches, the amount of mucus increases, and in the days around ovulation, it becomes clear and stretchy and can be detected by the woman if she puts a finger into the entrance of the vagina. Following ovulation, the production of mucus declines and the vaginal entrance becomes dry again.

If a woman is using this method as a means of family planning, she examines her vaginal entrance each day for the presence of mucus, and if she finds it, avoids sexual intercourse. However, vaginal wetness occurs for other reasons as well as discharge of cervical mucus, especially during sexual arousal, and the recognition of the 'dangerous days' may be difficult. This may mean that the couple avoid sexual intercourse on more days than are necessary to avoid conception; or they take a chance. In the reported studies of women who used the mucus method (also called the ovulation method or the Billing's method), between 15 and 25 in every 100 became pregnant in the first year of use, mostly because they failed to abstain from sex when they detected mucus, and others gave up the method.

For motivated couples, who choose not to use, or are prohibited from using, other methods of contraception, the mucus method has a definite place in family planning, provided that the couple abstain from sexual intercourse when any wet, lubricative and stretchy mucus is detected.

Natural family planning: the sympto-thermal method

With this method of contraception, the woman records her menstrual cycles for 6 months, and calculates the 'safe' days (see *Natural family planning: the calendar method). Sexual intercourse is permitted from menstruation until the last safe day before *ovulation. As an added protection against an unwanted pregnancy, she also checks her basal body temperature each day (the temperature on waking) and only resumes sexual intercourse after the basal body temperature has been raised for three consecutive days. Symptoms of breast pain, changes in her cervical mucus, or the occurrence of *mittelschmerz are also noted.

An unexpected pregnancy occurs each year in 11 out of every 100 women who use this rather complicated method of birth control. The drop-out rate is fairly high, particularly among younger couples and those who want to have regular and frequent sexual intercourse.

Natural family planning: the calendar method

This is a method of avoiding pregnancy in which the woman charts her menstrual cycles over a period of 6 months. She then calculates the estimated time of *ovulation in each cycle by assuming it to be 14 days before the next menstruation. Sexual intercourse is unlikely to be followed by pregnancy if it is avoided during the 3 days before and the 3 days after ovulation. By referring to the chart the woman can calculate which days are 'safe' for her. As many women have cycles of variable length, the number of safe days in a cycle are correspondingly reduced, so that sexual intercourse has to be avoided for many days.

The chart on the following page shows a woman's cycles for six months. On the basis of her cycle her 'at risk' period extends from day 9 to day 21. The additional use of the mucus method enables the length of abstinence to be shortened.

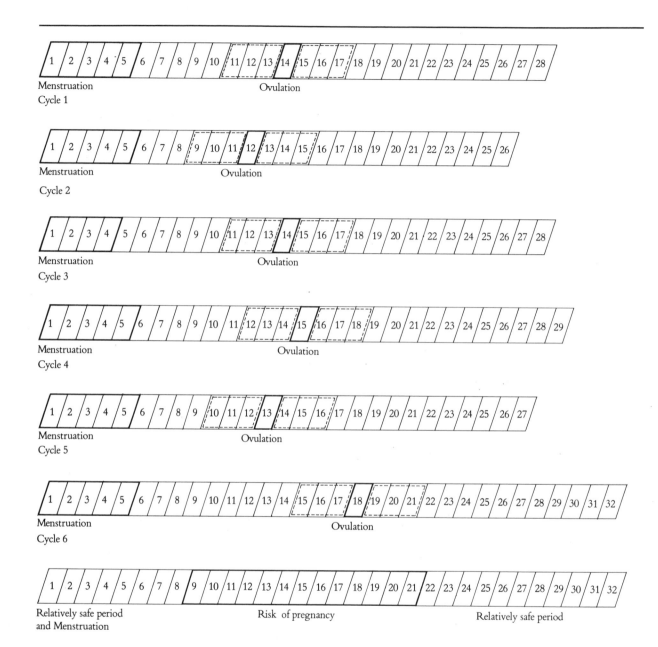

Menstruation Cycle 1 — Ovulation

Menstruation Cycle 2 — Ovulation

Menstruation Cycle 3 — Ovulation

Menstruation Cycle 4 — Ovulation

Menstruation Cycle 5 — Ovulation

Menstruation Cycle 6 — Ovulation

Relatively safe period and Menstruation — Risk of pregnancy — Relatively safe period

Neural tube defects

Early in the development of the embryo, the neural tube (which becomes the spinal cord and brain) lies in a groove extending along the back of the embryo. The two edges of the groove grow inwards and fold towards each other, fusing by the 6th week of pregnancy and covering the spinal cord. Occasionally, the headward part of the groove fails to close, with the result that the skull does not form and the brain is left exposed. This condition is called anencephaly. The groove may also fail to close at the lower (rear) end of the neural tube. This exposes the spinal cord in the area of the lower back, when the condition is called spina bifida. The spinal cord may be covered with its membranes, which bulge through the gap (a meningocele), or the nervous tissue itself may protrude (a myelomeningocele). The latter condition is more common.

An anencephalic baby can only live a few days, and is often born dead. If the baby has only a meningocele, surgery will cure the condition, but if the baby has an open spina bifida lesion containing nervous tissue the outlook is poor. The baby may have paralysed legs, hydrocephalus ('water on the brain'), or bladder involvement, which means that the child will be permanently incontinent. Full assessment soon after birth will enable the doctors to decide if surgery is feasible to give the baby a chance of a relatively normal life. If this is not considered possible, then surgery is not performed and the baby is nursed until it dies, which usually occurs from meningitis within 6 weeks.

Open neural tube defects (anencephaly and spina bifida) affect about 4 in every 1000 fetuses and can be diagnosed between the 14th and 18th week of pregnancy by tests on the mother's blood and on the amniotic fluid to measure a substance called alpha-fetoprotein. Raised levels of this substance indicate an open neural tube lesion. ★Ultrasound may also be used to help in the diagnosis but an ★amniocentesis may be necessary to measure the level of alpha-fetoprotein in the amniotic fluid before a firm diagnosis is made. If an open neural tube defect is found, the options are discussed with the parents, who can decide whether they wish to have the pregnancy terminated.

Nipple discharge

Nipple discharge which is watery, blood-stained, or thick may occur in a woman who is not pregnant. The woman should visit a doctor, who will examine the breasts to determine whether the discharge is due to a benign breast condition or to ★breast cancer.

A few pregnant women develop a brownish-red or chocolate-coloured discharge from their nipples in late pregnancy or in the first days after childbirth. Occasionally it occurs some months after childbirth. The cause of the discharge is not known. There is no treatment, and the woman can continue to breast-feed if she wishes. Should the discharge persist for 4 weeks or so, she should visit a doctor, although it is unlikely that any disease is present.

Other women find that milk seeps from their nipples spontaneously or when their breasts are fondled, at a time when they are not breast-feeding. This condition, known as 'inappropriate lactation' or ★galactorrhoea, may be associated with ★amenorrhoea. It should be investigated, which will include measurement of the hormone ★prolactin in a blood sample and an X-ray of the pituitary area of the skull. The purpose of the investigations is to find out if there is a tumour in the pituitary gland. If there is no tumour but the milk discharge worries the woman, or if she wishes to have regular menstruation so that it is possible for her to become pregnant, ★bromocriptine may be prescribed.

Non-consummation

The term 'non-consummation' when applied to a relationship between a man and a woman indicates that there has been no penetration of the vagina by the penis. This may occur because the man is unable either to achieve an erection at all or to achieve an erection for long enough for his penis to be inserted in the vagina (erectile failure). It may occur because the woman suffers from the condition called ★vaginismus, when she involuntarily contracts the muscles surrounding the vaginal entrance so strongly that penetration by the penis is impossible. Non-consummation of a relationship may occur in the absence of vaginismus because the woman fears injury to herself, or she may be ashamed of or ignorant about the anatomy of her vagina.

Non-consummation
Non-gonococcal urethritis
Non-specific vaginitis

Vaginismus is the most common cause of non-consummation. The woman often enjoys cuddling but is hesitant to caress the man's penis. If he tries to insert a finger into her vagina, or attempt *sexual intercourse, the muscles around her vagina go into spasm, and sometimes she draws her thighs together. A similar spasm occurs if a doctor attempts to perform a vaginal examination. Although a number of women who suffer from vaginismus believe they have an abnormally small vagina, or are 'small made', this is untrue. There is no such thing as a small vagina in a woman who has not undergone vaginal surgery, and there is no place for surgery in the treatment of vaginismus. The underlying cause is a lack of knowledge about the anatomy of the vagina, and a fear of penetration. The latter may be due to an upbringing which stressed the 'dirty' nature of sex. Most sexual matters, if discussed at all, were treated negatively and prefaced by 'don'ts': 'Don't let a boy touch you down there', 'Don't go out with boys', and so on. Fear of penetration may arise from inaccurate information obtained from other girls. These negative attitudes to sex induce the woman to fear that sexual intercourse will be painful.

Treatment is not complicated, but may require several sessions with a trained counsellor. In these sessions the woman's genital anatomy is explained, and the doctor asks if he may examine her vagina with his finger. During this session, the woman inspects her genitals in a mirror and is invited to feel inside her vagina with her finger. When she is comfortable about doing this, she may allow a doctor to introduce a *speculum into her vagina, or she may be provided with a set of graded plastic dilators, ranging in size from a pencil to a penis. She learns to insert these, and when she finds that she can do it painlessly and without her muscles going into spasm she is given permission to try sexual intercourse. Her partner is usually involved in the re-education programme. His attitudes to sexuality are discussed, and his approach to the woman is assessed. Some men are ignorant about sexual intercourse, or are insensitive to the woman's needs. Once the woman has lost her fear of penetration, intercourse may be attempted. The couple learn that they must spend time in *sexual pleasuring before penetration is attempted, so that the woman becomes relaxed, her vagina becomes wet, and she is receptive.

Non-gonococcal urethritis

Non-gonococcal urethritis (NGU) – infection of the urethra – is now the most common sexually transmitted disease found among men. The man complains of a burning sensation on passing urine and often has a discharge from his urethra. In about 50 per cent of cases the disease is due to a microbe called *Chlamydia* which lives inside cells. *Chlamydia* urethritis may persist for months.

It has been reported that about 70 per cent of the female contacts of men with chlamydial NGU are infected. Because of this the sexual partner or partners of a man who has NGU should be treated regardless of whether she has symptoms of urethritis. A course of antibiotics is prescribed (usually tetracycline or erythromycin) which the woman has to take for 3 weeks.

Non-specific vaginitis

Non-specific vaginitis is the name given to an infection which gives rise to vaginal discharge and is caused neither by *trichomonad infection nor by *candidiasis. Usually the discharge is thin, greyish in colour, has a disagreeable odour, and may cause itching. It is thought to be due to the interaction between two kinds of bacteria which normally live in the vagina: one type called *Gardnerella*, and others called anaerobes which grow in the absence of oxygen. The treatment is the same as that for *trichomonad infection, but it is not always successful and other treatments may be needed.

Obesity

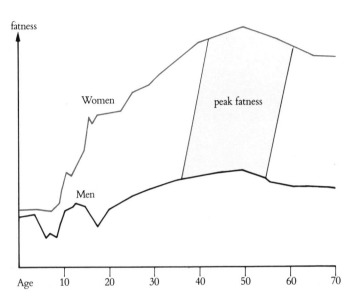

An obese person has an abnormally high proportion of body fat, which is usually the result of over-eating over a period of time. The overweight person and the obese person can be distinguished by dividing the body weight (in kilogrammes) by the height² (in metres). This gives an index which ranges from 20 to more than 40. The weight/height² or 'body-mass' index which defines obesity is 30 or more. If a person's body-mass index is greater than 30, then there is greater risk to life. By the age of 40, about 12 per cent of

men and at least 16 per cent of women are obese.

The causes of obesity are complex. Each obese person has taken in more energy into her body (by food and drink) than she has used for maintaining her bodily functions, for repair, and for exercise. The excess energy is converted into fat. Some obese people do very little exercise and consequently do not use up energy for that purpose. Other obese people are more efficient in their use of energy, using less than other people doing similar activities, and so have more energy to convert to fat. While other obese people are less efficient in *losing* energy as heat loss through their skin.

Obesity can be treated. Dieting is the safest and most appropriate way of losing weight. 'Crash diets' and 'gimmicky diets' should be avoided as they are relatively ineffective and may be dangerous. A balanced diet, which provides about 2.1 megajoules (500 kcals) a day *less* than is needed for bodily functions, will result in the loss of 0.5 kg of fat a week; this is the ideal rate at which to lose weight. Several diets of this type have been devised. In addition, motivation is needed to help the woman keep to the diet. There is considerable evidence to show that a woman who joins one of the self-help groups such as TOPS (Take Off Pounds Sensibly) or WWI (Weight Watchers International) is more likely to achieve her desired weight loss and to maintain her lower weight. Exercise also helps in weight loss and is beneficial, but only if the woman enjoys exercise.

Oedema in pregnancy

In pregnancy, water is retained in the tissues of the woman's body, the quantity varying between 1000 and 2500 ml. In late pregnancy, the flow of blood from the lower limbs is impeded by the enlarged uterus, which increases the pressure in the leg veins and leads to further accumulation of fluid in the tissues. About one pregnant woman in 3 develops swelling of the ankles and lower legs towards evening, a condition known as

oedema. This form of oedema is without significance, and the treatment is for the woman to put her legs up. Oedema may also occur in association with ★pre-eclampsia, when it becomes more important. Often the first sign of this form of oedema is a weight gain in excess of 1 kg a week, which does not respond to dieting. This is why a woman is weighed at each antenatal visit, so that her weight gain can be carefully monitored.

Oestriol tests

During pregnancy, the levels of the female sex hormone oestriol in the woman's blood and urine rise. Oestriol is produced from simple chemicals in a pregnant woman's body, and the fetus is involved in some of the chemical stages required for its composition. This led to the suggestion that the levels of oestriol in the woman's blood or urine would to some extent reflect the condition of the fetus. If the fetus was malnourished or its bodily processes were impaired, the level of oestriol in the mother would fall. A test is carried out to measure the level of oestriol in the mother's blood or urine (collected over 24 hours) several times a week. As the level of the hormone varies considerably from day to day, the test only becomes significant if the fall in the level of oestriol persists over several days. This limits its value, and in many hospitals the test has been superseded by recording the *Fetal Kick Count or by performing *cardiotocography.

Oestrogens

Oestrogens are the principal female sex hormones and are produced in the ovaries following stimulation by hormones from the pituitary gland (see *Menstruation, normal). Oestrogens are first produced in any quantity after *puberty, and the amount produced in the body declines markedly after the *menopause.

The effect of oestrogen is to stimulate the growth of the tissues of the female genital tract. This results in the vagina developing more and the uterus becoming bigger. Oestrogen also leads to the growth of the breasts and nipples and stimulates the deposition of fat on the hips, which gives a woman her characteristic shape. In the absence of any significant amounts of oestrogen at puberty, which occurs in a condition called *Turner's syndrome, the girl fails to develop breasts, and her genital organs remain infantile. However, treatment with tablets of synthetic oestrogen leads to the normal development of her breasts and genitals.

Synthetic oestrogens are used in the contraceptive *pill, in the treatment of menopausal symptoms, and in some cases they are also used to regulate irregular menstrual periods.

Older primigravida

A woman who becomes pregnant for the first time when she is aged 30 or more is referred to as an 'older primigravida'. This is an improvement on the term 'elderly primigravida' which was used until recently. Current statistics show that fewer than 15 per cent of women wait until the age of 30 to give birth to their first child. In past years obstetricians expressed concern about delay in childbearing. Today with better health and hygiene and with better obstetric services, the effect of the mother's age on obstetric performance is less. There is a slightly higher chance that an older primigravida will develop a raised *blood pressure during pregnancy and will be delivered by *Caesarean section. However, if she seeks *antenatal care as early as possible in pregnancy, and attends regularly, few problems arise either in pregnancy or during childbirth.

Oligohydramnios

In a few pregnant women, the amount of *amniotic fluid is much smaller than normal. The condition is called oligohydramnios, and if it occurs, the baby is compressed by the uterus instead of being able to swim freely in its water-filled capsule, the amniotic

Oligohydramnios
Ophthalmia of the newborn
Oral sex
Orgasm, failure to reach

sac. The compression, over a period of time, may be followed by serious consequences to the fetus, leading to deformities of its spine, to club foot, and occasionally to damage of the lung.

Oligohydramnios is rare, and can be due to damage to or absence of kidneys in the baby, so that it is unable to pass urine. The baby is usually born prematurely and does not survive.

Ophthalmia of the newborn

If a pregnant woman's cervix harbours gonococci (the bacteria which cause *gonorrhoea), the baby's eyes may be infected as he passes through the *birth canal. The condition only occurs rarely, but in some countries, such as the United States, prophylactic eyedrops are put routinely in the eyes of every newborn baby. Usually 1% silver nitrate is chosen, but some doctors use penicillin eyedrops. Silver nitrate, however, can cause marked irritation of the eyes and it is probably better to avoid prophylactic eyedrops and to treat any baby who develops a gonorrhoeal eye infection in the first 10 days of life. If untreated, gonococcal ophthalmia leads to blindness.

Oral sex

Oral sex includes licking or sucking a man's penis (fellatio) and licking a woman's clitoral area (cunnilingus). Oral sex is used by many couples as a means of *sexual pleasuring, and often the man or woman wishes the partner to continue until orgasm is reached. As only 50 per cent of women regularly reach orgasm during *sexual intercourse, many wish their partner to help them reach orgasm by cunnilingus, and over 90 per cent of women will do so. The strength of an orgasm reached during oral sex is no less intense than that reached during intercourse.

If the woman is sucking the man's penis he may ejaculate semen into her mouth.

Although the taste is rather acrid, it will cause no harm if she swallows the semen. Some men are unwilling to lick a woman's clitoris because they believe that the genital area is 'dirty', whereas it is in fact cleaner than the mouth.

In pregnancy, some women prefer cunnilingus because sexual intercourse is uncomfortable. There is no danger to either the woman or the fetus, provided that the man does not blow into her vagina.

Oral sex is a normal and appropriate way of sexual pleasuring. It can be enjoyed if both partners wish it, and if neither has a religious or moral objection.

Orgasm, failure to reach

About 50 per cent of women are unable to reach orgasm during *sexual intercourse, either because the man reaches orgasm too quickly or because he does not stimulate the woman in the way she prefers. Another 40 per cent of women are able to reach and enjoy orgasm if their clitoral area is stimulated directly, either by masturbating, by their partner's fingers or tongue (*oral sex), or by means of a *vibrator. Many women who learn to reach orgasm in these ways subsequently find that they can reach orgasm during sexual intercourse. These figures show that at least 90 per cent of women can reach orgasm by one means or another, and only 10 per cent consistently fail to do so (anorgasmia). It should be stressed that reaching orgasm is only one aspect of a sexual relationship. Women who fail to do so consistently should not feel that they are freaks or that they are at fault in some way. These women may receive much pleasure from cuddling and from the feeling generated when their partner reaches orgasm.

Osteoporosis

Osteoporosis is a condition in which over the years the bones become less dense, contain less calcium, and fracture more easily. It is the most common bone disease and particularly affects women who have passed the *menopause. The fact that the bones are less strong may not in itself cause any trouble, but often a fracture occurs either of the forearm or of the hip, or else a vertebra collapses, causing back pain. Fractures occur because, over the years, the bone tissue is lost at the rate of about 1 per cent each year. When the bones become brittle, fractures are likely. This usually occurs after the age of 60.

The development of osteoporosis is complex. It is related to ageing, lack of exercise, lack of calcium in the diet (or, more probably, a reduced ability to absorb calcium from the food), and lack of the female sex hormone *oestrogen. Oestrogen is only secreted in small amounts after the menopause.

In its early stages, osteoporosis is without symptoms, though some women complain of backache or spasm of the back muscles. Later, the woman may develop a 'dowager's hump', as a vertebra collapses, and she may become less tall, shrinking in height. In these early stages, further progress of the disease can be prevented in several ways. Firstly, women who have passed the menopause should take more exercise than many do. Secondly, they should include more calcium in their diet, either by eating more cheese or by taking more milk, as milk drinks or used in cooking. They should also take a calcium tablet (1000 mg) each night. Thirdly, oestrogen may be prescribed in tablet form as this prevents further bone loss. The use of oestrogen is controversial as it may increase the chance of developing cancer of the uterine lining (*endometrial cancer).

Hormone treatment is more efficient than calcium treatment, but the choice of treatment will depend on the individual needs and condition of each woman, as assessed in discussion with her doctor.

Ovarian tumours

Ovarian tumours are usually cystic, forming an ovarian cyst in nearly all cases and only 5 per cent being solid tumours. An ovarian cyst is a sac filled with fluid which grows on or in the ovary. Over 95 per cent of ovarian tumours are not cancerous, but a solid tumour is more likely to be malignant. Most ovarian tumours produce no symptoms and are found when a woman is examined vaginally during a gynaecological check-up. Some ovarian cysts alter the pattern of the menstrual cycle and this may lead to a diagnosis. Small ovarian cysts (less than 5 cm) may be observed without further treatment for one or two months, as many disappear in this time, but large ovarian cysts require surgery. The diagnosis may be helped by means of *ultrasound or X-ray. In younger women of childbearing age, the surgeon usually tries to 'shell' the cyst or tumour out of the ovary, which he then reconstructs. In women over 45, it is usual to remove the whole ovary which contains the tumour. If *ovarian cancer* is detected, the surgeon usually removes both the ovaries and the uterus, in order to prevent the cancer spreading further. If the ovarian cancer is advanced when first detected, as it very often is, *chemotherapy may be the suggested treatment after surgery.

Ovaries, removal of

Occasionally the ovaries of a woman under the age of 50 have to be removed because of disease, and in older women the ovaries are sometimes removed when a *hysterectomy is carried out. The reason for removal in both cases is to avoid ovarian cancer. If possible, the ovaries of a young woman should not be removed as this results in severe symptoms

Ovaries, removal of
Ovulation
Ovulation pain and bleeding
Oxytocics

of the *menopause. In the case of older women, although ovarian cancer is prevented, the absence of the ovaries prevents the formation of certain substances which enable other tissues of the body to produce oestrogen. The doctor and the woman should discuss the matter before surgery and reach an acceptable decision. Younger women will require *hormone replacement therapy, as do many older women.

Ovulation

Ovulation is the process whereby an egg (or ovum) which has developed in an *egg follicle, under the influence of the pituitary hormones, is expelled from the follicle and taken into the Fallopian tube. The time of ovulation during the menstrual cycle assumes importance if the couple are infertile, and also if one of the *'natural' methods of family planning is used. In all ovulatory menstrual cycles ovulation occurs 13 to 15 days (usually 14 days) before the first day of the next menstrual period. As this is a retrospective way of determining ovulation, other methods are used to pinpoint it prospectively. One method is for the woman to keep a chart of her temperature taken each day before rising. In ovulatory menstrual cycles, the body temperature rises by 0.3°C in the second half of the cycle, and ovulation can be estimated to occur as the temperature rise happens. Another method is for the woman to check her vaginal secretions each day. Around the time of ovulation they become clear, easily stretched, and profuse. A more accurate method is to measure the level of the female sex hormone *oestrogen in the urine or blood each day for about 7 days around the middle part of the menstrual cycle. The amount of oestrogen peaks suddenly about 12 to 24 hours before ovulation occurs. Alternatively, the pituitary hormone, *luteinizing hormone (LH), is measured; it peaks at 12 to 24 hours before ovulation.

Ovulation does not occur from alternate ovaries each month; chance determines which egg follicle will grow most quickly, so that chance also determines from which ovary the egg is expelled.

Ovulation pain and bleeding

A few women complain of pain in the lower abdomen which occurs at mid-cycle, halfway between the menstrual periods. The pain lasts a few hours, and a small amount of blood may be noticed at the entrance to the vagina. The condition is caused by *ovulation. Just before the egg is expelled from the ovary into the Fallopian tube, it stretches the surface of the ovary and this causes the pain (*mittelschmerz).

Oxytocics

Oxytocics are a group of drugs which, when injected or given by mouth, make the uterus contract. Three main oxytocics are available: ergometrine, which is extracted from a fungus which grows on rye; a laboratory-made oxytocin (Syntocinon or Pitocin), which resembles the natural oxytocin made in the pituitary gland; and prostaglandin.

Oxytocic drugs are used to initiate labour, and to increase the strength of the uterine contractions. Prostaglandin can be given as vaginal tablets or intravenously, while oxytocin has to be given by an intravenous infusion. Ergometrine is never used as it causes uterine spasm too easily.

Oxytocics are also used to prevent, or to treat, haemorrhage after childbirth (*postpartum haemorrhage) when ergometrine is usually given, but oxytocin may be chosen, and often the drugs are mixed in one injection (Syntocinon). This technique has reduced the risk of postpartum haemorrhage to less than 2 per cent.

Painful intercourse

Painful intercourse (dyspareunia) is a symptom and may be due to a local condition of the woman's external genitals, vagina, or pelvis, or may occur for psychological reasons. The most common local conditions are vaginal inflammation and conditions of the external genitals; some women have painful intercourse for weeks or months following stitching required to treat a *perineal tear or an *episiotomy after childbirth. When the pain is felt deep in the pelvis as the woman's partner thrusts strongly with his penis, the cause may be *pelvic infection or *endometriosis.

In most cases, dyspareunia is due to a psychological fear of being hurt during sexual intercourse, or ignorance about the *anatomy of the internal genitals, or to a belief that sex is 'dirty'. Some women who find intercourse painful believe the vagina is too small for the man's penis. The vagina is never too small, unless it has been damaged or has been operated upon inexpertly. In extreme cases, the woman is unable to let the man even touch her genitals. If he does, the muscles surrounding her vagina go into spasm, a condition called *vaginismus which prevents penetration.

Treatment of painful intercourse is to correct the physical problem, if one has been found, and to treat the psychological problem by explanation, sympathetic counselling, or psychotherapy from an experienced sexual counsellor.

Paracervical block

The nerves which carry painful sensations from the uterus pass through an 'exchange', which lies adjacent to the upper part of the cervix. If a local anaesthetic is injected into the area, most sensations of pain from the uterus are blocked. The injection is used for women who have an *induced abortion, so that the fetus and placenta can be sucked out of the uterus painlessly. It is also used occasionally to reduce the pain of childbirth, although it has largely been replaced by *epidural anaesthesia.

Parenthood, adjustment

It is well known that in most societies, the birth of a baby disturbs the life of the mother far more than that of the father, and many women have problems in adjusting to parenthood. Most women are brought up to believe that they should simultaneously be good housekeepers, excellent lovers, and experienced mothers. Yet when a woman finds herself caring for a newborn baby, its persistent demands on her energy, time, and emotions, may cause her considerable stress. This is often intensified by the modern 'nuclear' family and the tendency for close family members to live at some distance from each other. The pressures on the new mother increase as she realizes that she has sole responsibility for a small infant who needs – and demands – constant attention. The baby's crying, often for so little apparent cause, is wearing, she suffers from broken sleep, adding fatigue to her feelings of maternal inadequacy. The change in her relationship with her husband or partner can be an additional emotional burden, especially if he does not take an active part in caring for the baby. The woman finds that she is unable to look after the house properly as the baby takes up so much of her time, which makes her feel guilty.

The whole burden of physical and emotional readjustment may give rise to periods of uncontrollable weeping, or episodes of anger followed by sadness. Some women, while adjusting to parenthood, do outrageous things which do not fit with their characters. Others develop *postpartum depression. Adjustment to being a parent becomes easier if the father takes his share of domestic duties, helps look after the baby, and is able to reassure the mother that she is loved and that she is coping. In addition, a sympathetic relative or a friend who is prepared to 'mother' the mother and to relieve her for periods of the responsibility of caring for the baby will help her adjust more easily to her new role.

Parity

Parity refers to the number of pregnancies which have reached a period when the baby could survive outside the mother's uterus. In other words it is said to be 'viable'. In many countries, viability is said to occur when the pregnancy has reached the 28th week. But in an increasing number of countries viability occurs when the pregnancy has reached the end of the 20th week. A nulliparous woman is one who has never completed a pregnancy to this stage, although she may have aborted previously. A primiparous woman is a woman whose pregnancy has reached viability. A multiparous woman is one who has given birth to a 'viable child' even if the baby was stillborn. To add to the complexity of the concept of parity, a woman's parity is not greater if a single baby, twins, or quads are born for parity refers to the viable *pregnancy*, not the number of babies in the uterus.

Partogram

A partogram is a graphic method of describing the progress of childbirth. The partogram is started on the woman's admission to hospital when several things are recorded. These include: the rate at which the baby's heart is beating; the position of the baby's head as assessed by palpating (feeling) the woman's abdomen; the frequency of the contractions; the woman's blood pressure and pulse rate.

A partogram is useful in that the progress of labour can be seen visually and action can be taken if the progress is slow (see ★Childbirth, labour). Most maternity hospitals and units today use partograms to record progress in labour.

Pedophilia

Strictly speaking, pedophilia means love for a boy, but the children involved may be female or male, so that a more appropriate definition is sexual desire with a child as its object. The reason why some adults enjoy sexual relations with a child is unclear. In some instances, the adult is over-anxious, insecure about his or her sexual 'performance', and therefore chooses an inexperienced, pliable partner. In other cases, the adult may believe in the myth that having sexual relations with a child will have a rejuvenating effect. Another factor may be the novelty of having a sexual relationship with an innocent, 'unspoiled' child.

Sexual contacts between adults and children involve caressing, stimulation of the penis or vulva by hand or mouth, and sex games, as much as sexual intercourse. In some cases, the relationship between the adult and the child is gentle and supportive. In others it is brutal and exploitative, and the child is sexually assaulted.

Children should feel sufficient confidence in their parents to be able to report to them any sexual advance made by an adult, whether a member of the family or a stranger. They should also be discouraged from accepting rides in cars or food of any sort from a stranger.

Pelvic congestion

Some women complain of a feeling of pressure in the pelvis, backache, and vague symptoms of being unwell. The pelvic discomfort may be felt throughout the menstrual cycle, but is often worse in the week before menstruation. Some women also complain of heavier periods. The symptoms are thought to be due to increased congestion of blood in the pelvic organs, especially the uterus and the veins which supply it.

Pelvic congestion is another example of a psychosomatic condition which is associated with emotional stress; this could be due to a poor relationship with a partner, anxiety about childbirth, concern about finances, or the woman's dissatisfaction with her life.

Because the symptoms suggest that the uterus is at fault, *hysterectomy is often advised. The results are not good. Initially, a woman with 'pelvic congestion' should seek the help of a psychologist or a psychiatrist, but only after she has been examined carefully by a doctor to make sure that no physical disease is present.

Pelvic examination

Women who attend a doctor because of gynaecological symptoms expect (and possibly fear) an internal examination, which is necessary so that the pelvic organs can be felt. The pelvic examination usually takes place with the woman lying on her back with her legs drawn up and separated. In the United States and some European countries, the woman's legs are supported by stirrups, and her body is covered with a sheet. The doctor first inspects the woman's external genitals, and then introduces a *speculum so that he may look at the cervix. Many women find this the most uncomfortable part of the examination, and a woman should expect to be told what sensations she may experience and what each step of the examination involves. She also has a right to expect that the speculum is warm – cold metal tends to make the muscles tense, which makes introduction of the instrument painful. The woman should relax her pelvic-floor muscles, by doing the opposite of what she does when she stops urinating.

In the final part of the examination, the doctor slowly inserts two of his fingers and feels for the uterus and the ovaries. This is not painful but can be uncomfortable, and the experience is made more pleasant if the doctor talks to the patient and explains what he is doing and what he hopes his examination will demonstrate.

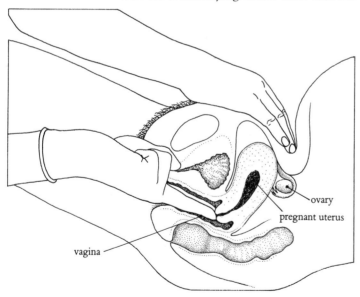

ovary

pregnant uterus

vagina

Pelvic infection

Pelvic infection, also known as pelvic inflammatory disease (PID), seems to be increasing in frequency. The woman has lower abdominal pain, may develop a fever, when examined vaginally complains of tenderness and pain, and the doctor may detect a tender swelling. PID follows infection with *gonorrhoea, following a spontaneous or

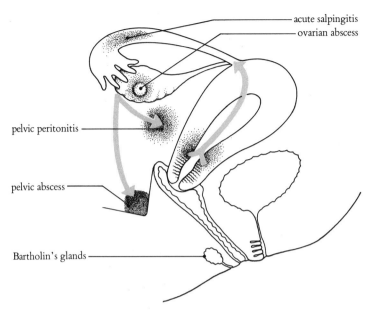

acute salpingitis
ovarian abscess
pelvic peritonitis
pelvic abscess
Bartholin's glands

induced *abortion, or after childbirth. In recent years, PID, following infection with a bacteria-like organism called *Chlamydia*, has become increasingly common. Like gonorrhoea, *Chlamydia* is sexually transmitted. It has also been observed that a woman who has used an *IUD has a slightly greater chance of developing PID. The diagnosis may be easy, but may be difficult, and at least 30 per cent of women treated for PID do not have any pelvic infection. Because of this, gynaecologists now frequently examine the pelvis with a *laparoscope before making a diagnosis, and at the same time take swabs from the inside of the abdomen for bacteriological examination. Treatment is to give an appropriate antibiotic, and analgesics to relieve the pain. Even when given good treatment, PID may be followed in some cases by *infertility and by a higher chance of *ectopic pregnancy if the woman conceives.

Pelvic pain

Chronic pelvic pain can be a most disturbing condition and affects an unknown number of women. The pain may be due to *pelvic infection, *endometriosis, or to bowel disease, but in most cases no physical cause can be found. In other words, it may be a psychosomatic condition. In most cases of unexplained pelvic pain, the doctor will take a very careful history and then inspect the pelvic organs using a *laparoscope, before diagnosing the pain as psychosomatic. Treatment depends on the cause: physical conditions are often corrected surgically, while psychosomatic pelvic pain requires supportive counselling and psychotherapy. Depression and *sexual problems which are not uncommonly found among women with chronic pelvic pain require treatment.

Perinatal mortality

The perinatal period extends from the 20th week of pregnancy to the end of the 4th week after childbirth. This period is the most hazardous for humans until they reach the age of 65! The hazard is determined by calculating the perinatal mortality rate.

The perinatal mortality has two components. First, fetal deaths (or stillbirths), that is the deaths before birth of all babies weighing more than 500 g, or whose gestation period (that is the duration in weeks since the mother's last period) exceeded 20 weeks. Second, neonatal deaths, that is babies born alive who die in the first 28 days of life.

The perinatal mortality rate is calculated as follows:

Fetal deaths + neonatal deaths per 1000 births

In some countries, only those babies dying in the uterus after the 28th week of pregnancy (late fetal deaths or stillbirths) and only those babies dying in the first 7 days of life are included. These deaths are added and the rate per 1000 births is calculated. This gives the basic or standard perinatal mortality rate.

In most developed nations the perinatal mortality rates have fallen considerably in the past thirty years. In England and Wales in the 1930s the standard perinatal mortality was 60 per 1000 births. Since 1940 it has fallen steadily and is now about 12 per 1000 births. In Australia the standard perinatal mortality in 1939 was 54 per 1000 births, by 1981 it had fallen to 10 per 1000 births. A similar fall is reported from the United States.

Within a country the perinatal mortality rate varies. It is three times as high in Social Classes IV and V in Britain compared with Social Class I, and similar findings have been reported from Australia, Scandinavia, and the United States. It is higher among women under the age of 17 or over the age of 35 and those who have had four or more previous children.

The decline in the perinatal mortality rate has occurred for several reasons: the change to smaller families; the availability and acceptance of *antenatal care; the improved care and supervision of childbirth; the provision of well-equipped, well-staffed, intensive neonatal units, where premature and sick babies can be given special care.

Today, in 98 out of 100 cases where the pregnancy has reached 20 weeks, the woman can expect that her baby will be born alive and will survive.

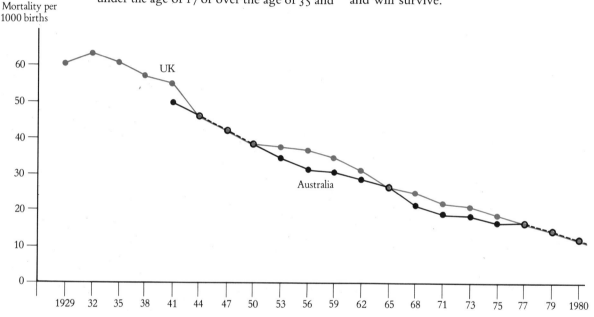

Perineal tear

The perineum is the area of tissue which lies between the vagina and the rectum. It is made up of muscle, covered on the outside by skin and on the inside by the mucous membrane surfaces of the vagina and the rectum. It is triangular in shape. During childbirth, the tissues of the perineum have to stretch to let the baby's head be born. As the tissues tend to be rather tense, perineal tears are common, at least among Western women. They are said to be less common among women in primitive societies, and this may be because they habitually squat, or

because childbirth is more 'natural'. Perineal tears are unusual in other animals, mainly because the fetal head of apes, monkeys, and other mammals is small and pointed, while a baby's head is relatively large and round.

Perineal tears can often be avoided if the birth is conducted slowly and carefully. In past years midwives were critized if the perineum was torn during childbirth. They were told to 'support the perineum' and did so, although often the skin remained intact but the muscles separated. If a tear occurs it may be small or may stretch into the woman's rectum. Left alone perineal tears heal, often painfully and inadequately. Modern obstetricians stitch a perineal tear once the baby and the placenta have been delivered. As the tear may have jagged edges, and the stitches are painful, many obstetricians prefer to make a deliberate incision into the perineum, as the baby's head stretches it, if they feel that a perineal tear is likely to occur. This is called an *episiotomy.

Petting

Petting is an American term for love-making which reaches, but stops short of, *sexual intercourse. Petting is as old as tribal society, and is practised by tribes as primitive as those of New Guinea, or by people with a culture as sophisticated as that of the United States. In Western countries, petting seems to be confined largely to adolescence. In 'light petting' or 'necking', the couple kiss passionately, their bodies (usually fully clothed) are in contact, but certain zones are 'forbidden' by the girl, who may refuse to allow her breasts to be caressed, and will not allow wandering hands to reach for her vulva. In 'heavy petting', passionate kissing, breast stimulation, caressing of the clitoris to orgasm and of the penis to ejaculation, and *oral sex, are accepted in varying degrees, but the girl remains a technical virgin, as she does not allow the man's penis to enter her vagina.

Petting plays an important role in the development of sexual behaviour as it offers the opportunity for exploration of the body and genitals, and for emotional interaction. The body exploration which petting permits is important, particularly for those people who obtain a great deal of pleasure from the sense of touch. Since this is conditioned by childhood learning, it is likely that men would be more willing to touch and would obtain more pleasure from touching if they were not taught to believe that touching is 'weak', 'feminine' and unmanly. Many women enjoy body contact for long periods of lovemaking before they want to have sexual intercourse, and many men would find that they too could obtain much sexual pleasure from touching their partner if they could learn to overcome the inhibitions they have about it.

Physical handicap and sexuality

Until recently it was assumed that physically handicapped people had no need to express their sexuality. This false and cruel opinion stemmed from the care-takers rather than the disabled. Physically disabled people have the right to sexual information, the right to receive sexual education, the right to express themselves sexually, the right to form sexual relationships, and the right to become parents. In women, the main physical handicaps that occur are due to cerebral palsy, spinal cord injury, blindness, deafness, deformities following *mastectomy and also gynaecological surgery, and, in later years, handicaps which develop with diabetes and arthritis.

The effect of these handicaps on the person's sexuality varies considerably, but most handicapped women are just as capable as any non-handicapped women in forming relationships and in expressing themselves sexually. Women with cerebral palsy can form warm relationships in spite of their disability; these enhance the woman's self-esteem and give greater meaning to her life. This is movingly demonstrated in the film *Like Other People*, made in the United Kingdom. A woman who has suffered a spinal cord injury usually has normal menstrual function, can conceive, and bear children. She no longer receives any sexual pleasure from stimulation of her clitoris and vagina, but continues to obtain pleasure from nipple or breast stimulation or by developing other erogenous areas; and she can share in and enjoy her partner's sexual pleasure. With a diminished emphasis on genital sex, the couple may derive greater pleasure than before from a wide range of sexual options, such as bodily *sexual pleasuring, touching, caressing, and *oral sex. Women who are blind from birth or childhood can also learn about sexuality, by using their developed sense of touch to achieve what sighted people do with their eyes.

The Pill

Over 50 million women use oral contraceptives to control their fertility. In the twenty-three years since the pill was first introduced in the United States in June 1960, it has been modified several times, and today's pill contains much lower amounts of the two hormones *oestrogen and *gestagen than the original oral contraceptives. Oral contraceptives are available in four formulations: the *combined* oestrogen-gestagen formulation in which a standard dose of each hormone is taken; the *sequential* pill in which a standard dose of oestrogen is taken daily, but the quantity of gestagen taken in the first 11 days is less than half that taken in the last 10 days; a *triphasic* product which reduces the level of gestagen still further; a *progestogen-only* formulation (Mini-pill). In most developed countries between 25 and 35 differently named oral contraceptives are available, which is confusing both to those providing the contraceptives and to women themselves, particularly as some of the pills with different names contain identical quantities of the two hormones. Even in the case of the other pills, the differences may be more apparent than real.

The pill has both benefits and disadvantages. The *benefits* include the fact that the pill is the most effective way of preventing an unwanted pregnancy in a sexually active woman; that women taking the pill have much less *dysmenorrhoea; that women who take the pill develop fewer *breast lumps. The *disadvantages* are connected with its real and supposed side-effects, as some of them may be due to anxiety induced by reading sensational articles about the pill, or to guilt about using it. A few women become depressed when taking the pill; and a few have a rise in blood pressure. Menstruation tends to become lighter and the blood may change in colour to a dirty brown. Some women have an increased vaginal discharge, and a few find that they are less aroused sexually. The principal concern about the pill is that it increases a woman's chance of developing a clot in a vein (*venous thrombosis), a heart attack, or a stroke. These are very uncommon, however, and affect about 8 in every 100000 pill-users. They are more likely to occur in women who are over 35, overweight, and who smoke; it is likely that smoking is the main cause of these conditions, not the pill.

Before being prescribed the pill, a woman should be examined vaginally and her blood pressure taken. Women who have a history of clots in veins, heart attacks, or stroke should use another contraceptive method. Women who have liver disease, blood disease, severe migraine, or high blood pressure should also be advised to choose another form of contraception. Usually a woman is prescribed a pill containing the lowest dose of hormones (the low-dose or the triphasic formulation), and if this does not suit her, because her menstrual periods become erratic, a pill containing a higher dose of hormones is chosen.

The *Mini-pill is used for some women who cannot tolerate oral contraceptives containing oestrogen, or who should not use them, for example breast-feeding women, as their milk supply may be reduced. The Mini-pill is taken at the same time each day. It is not as effective in preventing pregnancy as the pill and is associated with a rather high frequency of 'breakthrough' bleeding. For these reasons its use is limited.

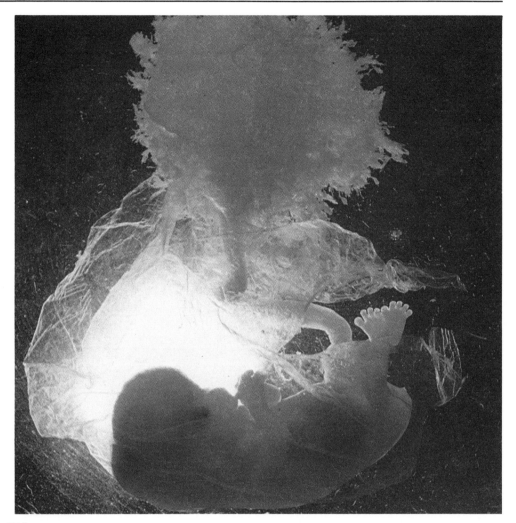

Placenta

The placenta (or afterbirth) is formed from part of the fertilized egg, and acts as a functional union between mother and baby. The organ is bathed by the mother's blood on one side, and by the *amniotic fluid on the other. It is made up of finger-like processes of cells, which join to give it a tree-like structure. The placenta acts as an organ of respiration and excretion for the fetus, performing the function of its lungs and its kidneys. Oxygen in the mother's blood is taken up by the placental cells and passes into the blood of the fetus. Waste products from the fetus are discharged into the mother's blood through the placenta. In addition, other important nutrients are extracted from the mother's blood and transferred to the fetus. The placenta produces and elaborates various hormones, including *oestrogen, *progesterone, and chorionic gonadotrophin. As the placenta is formed from genes derived from both parents, it might be expected that the mother's immune system would seek to destroy it, as it does other 'foreign' organs, such as kidney and heart transplants. It is unclear why the placenta is not rejected by the mother, but it is likely that the 'antigen sites' on the surface of the placental cells which are bathed by the mother's blood are coated with a substance which makes the body accept it.

Polycystic ovary

A few women whose menstrual periods have become scanty or have ceased, who are infertile, who have excess body hair, and who may be obese, have a condition called the polycystic ovarian syndrome in which the ovaries become larger and contain a number of cysts of various sizes. The condition is due to an imbalance of the pituitary hormones which control *ovulation. The diagnosis may be easy, or may have to be made with the use of a *laparascope and by measuring the amount of the hormone testosterone in a sample of blood. The woman may choose not to have any treatment at all or she may wish to have one or more of her complaints treated.

Polyhydramnios

This is a condition of pregnancy in which the amount of *amniotic fluid exceeds 3 litres. It has several causes, including fetal malformations, tumours of the placenta, and twins. Twins, especially identical (uniovular) twins, are the most common cause. Fetal malformations, especially *neural tube defects and a blockage of the gullet which prevents the baby swallowing, are the next most frequent causes. When a doctor detects polyhydramnios an *ultrasound picture is usually taken to discover if there is a *multiple pregnancy or if the baby is malformed.

Generally the fluid accumulates slowly, causing an abnormally large uterus, but occasionally it accumulates very rapidly. This causes the woman severe abdominal pain, breathlessness, and palpitations. Treatment depends on the severity of the symptoms. If they are marked, an *amniocentesis is carried out to draw off the fluid: but often this precipitates labour.

Post-maturity

Over 90 per cent of women give birth within 2 weeks of the estimated date of delivery. This is determined by noting the date of the start of the woman's last menstrual period, and the regularity of her menstrual cycle, and supplementing this information, if need be, by an *ultrasound examination made between the 10th and 14th week or between the 16th and 20th week of pregnancy. In 5 per cent of women, the pregnancy continues for 2 weeks past the estimated date of delivery (prolonged pregnancy). As the pregnancy becomes post-dated, or post-mature, the risk to the baby doubles. In these cases, it is usual to check the woman each week and to monitor the fetus by *cardiotocography. If the baby's head is engaged in the pelvis and the cervix is soft, labour may be *induced by amniotomy; but if these conditions do not apply and the cardiotocograph shows the baby to be at significant risk of dying, the obstetrician may decide that a *Caesarean section is necessary, after discussion with the woman and her partner.

Post-menopausal bleeding

If a woman who has passed the *menopause notices blood appearing at the entrance of her vagina, whether merely spotting or in larger amounts, she should seek immediate medical advice. The doctor will make a careful examination of the woman, including a *pelvic examination. He will take a *cervical smear, if this has not been taken recently, and he will recommend a *D and C. The purpose of carrying out these tests is to exclude the possibility of *cervical, *endometrial, and *ovarian cancer. However, most women who experience post-menopausal bleeding do not have cancer.

Postpartum haemorrhage

After childbirth it is normal for a woman to lose up to 500 ml of blood. If more blood is lost, this is called postpartum haemorrhage. Postpartum haemorrhage occurs in about 2 per cent of all births, and is more common if the mother has had twins, a prolonged labour, or has required deep anaesthesia. Most obstetricians prevent postpartum haemorrhage by giving the mother an injection of the drug *oxytocin as the baby's head is born. Oxytocin causes the uterus to contract and reduces the amount of blood lost.

Precocious puberty

A small number of girls become sexually mature before the age of 9. First their breasts develop, then hair appears on the pubis and in the armpits, and finally the girl menstruates. In most cases, the cause is familial, but investigations should be made to exclude hormone-producing *ovarian tumours, or a brain tumour. These include blood hormone assays, X-rays of the skull and bones, and a *pelvic examination under anaesthesia.

Pre-eclampsia

In about 7 per cent of all pregnant women, there is a rise in *blood pressure which takes the level of the diastolic pressure above 90 mm Hg (the diastolic pressure is the pressure between heart beats). The rise in blood pressure usually occurs after the 20th week, unless the woman has had a high blood pressure or renal (kidney) disease before pregnancy. High blood pressure which appears for the first time in the second half of pregnancy is called pre-eclampsia or, preferably, pregnancy-induced hypertension (PIH). In the past the illness was called toxaemia of pregnancy in the mistaken belief that it was caused by a toxin absorbed from the intestines. The cause of pre-eclampsia is unknown, but there is spasm of the blood vessels of the body. In mild cases, the spasm only produces the raised blood pressure (or hypertension); in more severe cases, the spasm also affects the kidneys, leading to a leak of *protein in the urine as well as hypertension; in the most severe cases, the woman may also start having fits. This condition is called *eclampsia.

If uncontrolled, pre-eclampsia is hazardous to the woman, as it may lead to eclampsia; and hazardous to the baby, who has a threefold risk of dying. The higher the blood pressure the greater the risk. Thus a woman's blood pressure is checked and a urine sample taken at each antenatal visit.

As the cause of pre-eclampsia is unknown, only the symptoms can be treated. Bed rest is usually recommended, as this improves the flow of blood through the uterus. If the diastolic blood pressure exceeds 110 mm Hg, or if fits appear likely, drugs are given to bring down the blood pressure. The welfare of the baby in the uterus is monitored (see *Fetal monitoring); and if its life becomes at risk, labour is *induced or a *Caesarean section is performed.

Most cases of pre-eclampsia complicate a first pregnancy, and the chance of it recurring in a second pregnancy is less than 5 per cent. The illness is self-limiting, and after delivery the symptoms disappear, causing no damage to the woman's body.

Pregnancy diagnosis

Pregnancy is diagnosed clinically if the woman has missed a period, if her breasts have become larger and tender, and if, on ★pelvic examination, the doctor finds that her uterus is enlarged. Some women are also nauseated or may need to pass urine frequently. Pregnancy can also be diagnosed by examining a sample of blood or urine from the woman. The test depends on the presence of the pregnancy hormone, human chorionic gonadotrophin (HCG) in the sample. The blood is tested in an instrument which measures the level of a part of HCG, called the beta-subunit, with great accuracy. With this technique, pregnancy can be diagnosed at the time of the missed period. The urine test is not accurate until about 40 days after the last menstrual period. A drop of urine is placed on a black slide, and a drop of anti-HCG is added. If the sample contains HCG, it will bind with the anti-HCG and form a complex. If the sample does not contain HCG, the anti-HCG is free. A drop of an indicator (white latex) coated with HCG is added to the sample. If the woman is pregnant, all the anti-HCG has been bound, and none is available to link with the latex coated with HCG, so the test solution stays in a milky condition. If the woman is not pregnant, however, the anti-HCG binds with the indicator and forms little white crystals which look like granulated sugar.

Pregnancy, minor complaints

Pregnant women suffer a number of complaints, which they consider too trivial to bring to the attention of their doctor, but which nevertheless cause them discomfort and anxiety. The most common of these 'minor' complaints are listed here.

Backache is common in late pregnancy. It is due to the alteration of the centre of balance by the growing fetus, which the woman counteracts by pushing her shoulders back. This puts a strain on her back muscles. In addition, low backache occurs from the relaxation of the sacroiliac and pubic ligaments due to pregnancy hormones.

Breathlessness Three-quarters of women experience breathlessness on exertion in the last 10 weeks of pregnancy. It is not due to disease, it will harm neither mother nor baby, and it disappears after childbirth.

Constipation The pregnancy hormones, probably ★progesterone, reduce the involuntary activity of the intestines, so that food and faeces travel more slowly through the intestines. This leads to constipation, which can be corrected by increasing the fibre in the diet (by eating wholemeal bread or taking bran), or by the intermittent use of laxatives, such as Senokot or Bisacodyl.

Fainting attacks, headaches, and palpitations are not unusual in pregnancy, and are due to the alterations in the woman's blood circulation.

★Haemorrhoids The pressure of the enlarging uterus on the blood returning from the lower bowel, together with constipation and straining to open the bowels, may cause haemorrhoids, especially during late pregnancy. If haemorrhoids occur and become painful, the woman should seek her doctor's advice.

Heartburn occurs quite commonly in late pregnancy, especially at night. It is due to a relaxation of the muscular valve which separates the oesophagus from the stomach. The relaxation permits the acid stomach contents to regurgitate into the oesophagus, where it causes a burning pain. There is no specific treatment, but eating small meals often and sleeping on two or more pillows is said to help the condition, as is the use of antacid tablets or mixtures.

Leg cramps occur in late pregnancy. Their cause is unknown. There is some (doubtful) evidence that milk intake exceeding a litre a day may be involved, so a pregnant woman should restrict her milk intake to 750 ml. It is also said that leg cramps at night are reduced if the foot of the bed is raised 25 cm.

Nausea, with or without vomiting, is common in early pregnancy but usually ceases by the 14th week. In some cases, nausea persists for much longer. Nausea is relieved if the woman eats small, non-fatty meals at frequent intervals. If this does not help, she may obtain anti-nausea tablets from her doctor.

Nose bleeds are not uncommon. They are due to the dilation of the blood vessels in the nose and the increased speed of the blood circulation. They are not a sign of high blood pressure.

*Pica This is a craving for strange foods which occurs in pregnancy; its cause is unknown.

Spongy gums A number of women find that their gums become swollen, spongy in appearance, and bleed easily, so that they seem to be affected by periodontal disease. The condition is not due to infection but to fluid retained in the cells of the gums. Unless the condition is painful, no treatment is needed. Mouth washes sometimes help to make the woman feel more comfortable but if in doubt a dentist should be consulted. The condition disappears following the birth of the baby.

Stretch marks These are fine, wavy, pinkish marks which appear on the lower abdomen or upper thighs of many pregnant women. They are not due to stretching but to the increased amount of a hormone in the tissues which 'fragments' the elastic fibres in the skin. There is no treatment. After pregnancy the marks fade and become faint.

Sweating In hot weather or after exertion many pregnant women sweat easily, particularly in the last weeks. The sweating is due to the dilated blood vessels in the skin, caused by pregnancy hormones. There is no specific treatment. If a pregnant woman finds sweating uncomfortable, she should try to take less exertion and bathe frequently.

Swollen ankles Swollen ankles occur frequently in the second half of pregnancy, usually in the evening. The swelling or

*oedema is often relieved if the woman puts her feet up, but if the oedema persists she should visit her doctor.

Urinary problems Many pregnant women feel the need to pass urine more frequently in early pregnancy and again in the last weeks. If this frequency is associated with pain or scalding on passing urine, a doctor should be informed as the woman may have urinary tract infection. About 50 per cent of women discover that they involuntarily pass a small amount of urine when they cough or laugh. There is no treatment and the 'incontinence' ceases after childbirth, particularly if the woman does *Kegel pelvic exercises.

*Urinary tract infection is more common in pregnancy and 5 per cent of pregnant women have a symptomless infection (called bacteriuria) before pregnancy. It is usual practice for the doctor to ask for a 'midstream' specimen of urine at the first antenatal visit. This is obtained by the woman cleaning the entrance to the vagina with a special swab, and collecting a specimen of urine once the stream is flowing. If bacteriuria is found, antibiotics are prescribed.

Later in pregnancy a few women develop fever, high backache, and scalding when they pass urine. If this occurs, a specimen of urine is examined to find if there is urinary infection, and it is treated.

*Vaginal discharge is most common in pregnancy. In many cases, the discharge is an exaggeration of normal vaginal moisture, but in a few it is due to *candida or *trichomonad infections. The discharge is associated with itching.

*Varicose veins In women who are predisposed to varicose veins, pregnancy may provoke their appearance, especially in the later months. The veins usually occur in the legs but veins in the woman's external genitals may become swollen. The symptoms are a feeling of heaviness in the legs and swelling of the ankles. Treatment is to keep the feet up as much as possible and, if necessary, to wear well-fitting elastic support stockings; the woman should put these on each morning before getting out of bed, when the veins are least obvious.

Premature labour

Labour is defined as premature (or preterm) if it begins before the 37th week of pregnancy, which would lead to the birth of a premature or ★preterm baby. In nearly half the cases of premature labour, no reason can be found. In most of the remaining cases, ★preeclampsia, twins, and diseases in the woman lead to the onset of premature labour. Drugs are now available which probably help to suppress the uterine contractions and prolong the pregnancy, but if the pregnancy has advanced to 34 weeks, and the woman is in a hospital which has a good neonatal care unit, it is better to avoid drugs and let the labour progress. Earlier in pregnancy, the risks of premature birth are greater and the drugs may be used. Currently, the ★beta-agonists (salbutamol and ritodrine) are favoured. These drugs reduce uterine activity but increase the heart rate causing palpitations, flushing, or headaches in many women, and their value is still being studied.

Premenstrual tension

Premenstrual tension (PMT) is not clearly defined, nor is it known what is the cause of a condition which affects more than 60 per cent of women between the ages of 20 and 45, and is severe in 20 to 40 per cent of cases. As nervous tension is only one of several complaints, the condition is more correctly called the premenstrual syndrome, but PMT is convenient and has been accepted into the language. PMT is a combination of emotional and physical symptoms, some of which occur with various degrees of severity during the last 7 to 14 days before menstruation and regress or disappear during menstruation. The most common symptoms are: *Irritability. Irrational anger. Short temper. Aggression. Nervous tension. Anxiety. Panic. Depression. Fatigue. Confusion.* ○ *Headaches. Dizziness.* ○ *Breast swelling, tenderness, and pain.* ○ *Abdominal bloating, tenderness. Weight gain. Backache. Swelling of legs, hands, occasionally the face.* ○ *Eating disturbances – increased appetite,* ★*'binge-eating', craving for sweets.* In spite of considerable research, the cause or causes of PMT remain obscure. Current research suggests that a disturbance of the neurotransmitters in the brain may be involved, and these may lead to disturbances in the level of female sex hormones circulating in the blood. The effect of treatment is variable, as placebos (sugar pills) relieve the symptoms in about 40 per cent of women, at least for a time. Some doctors prescribe vitamin B, others prescribe diuretics, and still others prescribe hormones, particularly injections of ★progesterone, ★gestagen in tablet form, or the contraceptive ★pill. In some cases, particularly if the main problem is breast tenderness or pain, ★bromocriptine has proved useful. Other doctors believe that PMT is a psychiatric condition and should be treated with anti-depressant or anti-anxiety drugs. None of the published results shows that any of the drugs tested is more effective than placebos. More careful and well-conducted research is required to understand a disorder which affects so many women and which is now recognized.

Prenatal influences

In many societies myths persist that a baby can be influenced by its mother's experiences during pregnancy. They developed to explain why some babies were born with ★congenital malformations. There is no truth that maternal impressions can affect an unborn baby. Firstly, the nervous and blood systems of the woman and the fetus are separate; secondly, the baby is completely formed by the 8th week of pregnancy; thirdly, most congenital defects are due to the transmission of abnormal genes, to environmental toxins, or to infections which can occur during pregnancy.

Preterm birth

In Western countries, a baby which weighs 2.5 kg or less and is born when the pregnancy is less than 37 weeks advanced, is said to be preterm (or premature). Preterm babies account for 8 per cent of all births, but for over three-quarters of all babies dying in the *perinatal period. If it were possible to prevent preterm births, most babies would survive. Some conditions predispose to preterm birth, but in many cases no cause for *premature labour and a preterm birth can be found. Certain factors are given in the following table (based on figures from the United Kingdom, United States, and Australia).

Cause of preterm birth	Per cent
No cause found	35-45
*Pregnancy-induced hypertension	10-20
*Multiple pregnancy	5-15
*Antepartum haemorrhage	5-10
*Congenital malformations	2-5
Diseases in the mother	2-5

It is difficult to prevent preterm births, although a nutritious diet before and during pregnancy, avoiding smoking, drugs, and excessive amounts of alcohol are said to help. The most effective way of reducing the risk of preterm birth is for the baby to be born in a hospital which has a well-equipped, well-run Intensive Neonatal Care Unit (INCU). This means that women who are at higher risk of having a preterm birth (as listed in the table, and women who have previously given birth to a preterm baby) should if possible be near a hospital which has an INCU during pregnancy. If this is not possible and the woman goes into premature labour, it is safer for the baby if she is transferred to a hospital with a unit while the baby is still in her uterus.

If the birth is preterm, the baby is likely to be nursed in an incubator and connected to various monitors, so that any irregularity of his breathing, his heart, or his blood electrolytes can be corrected quickly, and infection prevented.

In the past ten years increasing numbers of preterm babies have survived the dangerous weeks after birth and become healthy children. A baby weighing between 500 and 750 g at birth has a 28 per cent chance of surviving; one weighing 751 to 1000 g has a 50 per cent chance; a baby weighing 1001 to 1500 g has an 80 per cent chance; and one weighing 1501 to 2500 g has an 85 per cent chance of surviving.

Progesterone

Progesterone is the second female sex hormone produced in the ovary after *ovulation. It is secreted by the cells of the *egg follicle from which the egg has been expelled – the *corpus luteum. As its name implies, progesterone prepares the lining of the uterus (endometrium) for pregnancy, making it receptive to the fertilized egg.

The cells of the genital tract have many areas on their surfaces called receptor sites, and progesterone is able to bind to these sites and enter the cell. Within the cell it regulates the effect of *oestrogen. This is important as oestrogen stimulates both genital tract cells and breast cells to grow, and the regulating effect of progesterone controls their growth. This knowledge is used in treating some forms of advanced cancer, particularly *endometrial cancer and oestrogen-dependent *breast cancer; treatment is to give large doses of a synthetic progesterone (medroxy-progesterone acetate).

In pregnancy, large quantities of progesterone are secreted. The hormone relaxes smooth muscle – that is, the muscle of the uterus and of the bowel (which is why constipation is rather common in pregnancy). The hormone may also have a 'sedative' effect on brain cells, and account for the 'placidity' often found in pregnant women.

Prolactin

The hormone prolactin is secreted by cells in the pituitary gland and released into the blood. The secretion and release of prolactin are controlled by a substance formed in the hypothalamus. This substance, called dopamine, inhibits the synthesis and release of prolactin. In pregnancy, a steady rise in the blood level of prolactin occurs, and once the baby has been born, a rapid rise occurs, which is increased by suckling. The main function of prolactin is to stimulate the production of milk in the breasts, but it also acts on the ovary and the testis, suppressing their function.

A few women, who are not breast-feeding, stop having menstrual periods and often produce breast milk (★galactorrhoea). Investigations show that they have high blood levels of prolactin. The hormone comes from a tumour in the pituitary gland. Larger tumours require surgery, but the tiny (micro) tumours may be treated with ★bromocriptine which, like dopamine, prevents prolactin from being synthesized.

Prolapse

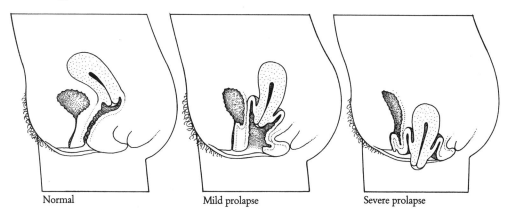

Normal   Mild prolapse   Severe prolapse

The word prolapse implies that the vagina has stretched so that its front wall bulges (a cystocele) or its back wall bulges (a rectocele) when the woman strains down, for example in opening her bowels. Usually, the supports of the uterus are stretched, so that it too 'prolapses' down when the woman strains, and the cervix of the uterus protrudes outside the vagina, like a questing nose.

Most prolapses occur in middle age or after the ★menopause as the strength of the supporting tissues decreases; but the damage which led to this usually occurred during childbirth, although a few childless women develop a prolapse.

Prolapse occurs less frequently today, as labours are not commonly permitted to last for more than 24 hours, without intervention to deliver the baby, and the second stage of

Prolapse can be or varying severity. The middle illustration shows the vaginal walls are lax and the womb has fallen slightly. The right-hand illustration shows a prolapse where the womb has protruded outside the body

labour (when the woman pushes) is not allowed to last for more than 2 hours. Women are also healthier and do not return to heavy work soon after childbirth.

Mild degrees of prolapse often respond to ★Kegel exercises, and if there are no other symptoms no further treatment is required. More severe degrees of prolapse are best treated by surgery. In a few elderly frail women, a supporting pessary may be placed in the vagina to hold the prolapsed tissue inside it and so avoid the need for surgery.

Prostaglandins
Protein in the urine
Psychological changes in pregnancy
Psychoprophylaxis

Prostaglandins

These are substances which are produced in many body tissues (especially the uterus) and which stimulate smooth muscle to contract. As the uterus is composed of smooth muscle, prostaglandins are effective in starting contractions. Prostaglandins are effective in inducing *abortions (particularly between the 15th and 20th weeks of pregnancy); in helping the uterus expel a dead fetus; and in the *induction of labour.

Prostaglandins can be given as vaginal tablets or pessaries; by injection into the space between the uterus and the *amniotic sac or into the amniotic sac; by injection into a vein or by mouth. A drawback to the use of prostaglandins is that they cause quite severe nausea, vomiting, and in some cases intestinal cramps and diarrhoea. The side-effects are reduced if prostaglandins are given into the vagina or the uterus.

Protein in the urine

The kidneys act as super-efficient filters, getting rid of waste products from the body, but retaining those substances the body needs. Protein, the substance the body uses for repair of its tissues, only appears in the urine if the kidney's filtering mechanism becomes defective. This may occur in kidney disease, in *pre-eclampsia during pregnancy (where spasm of the blood vessels supplying the kidney leads to temporary damage to its filter cells), and occasionally in some people when they stand for a long time. If protein is found in the urine, tests should be carried out to try to determine the cause.

Psychological changes in pregnancy

It is said that pregnancy and childbirth affect the father's life-style only marginally, but are turning-points in the life of a woman. For many women, pregnancy fulfills deep and powerful emotional needs, but it may also be a time of stress and readjustment. In the first weeks of pregnancy, the fetus may be perceived either as a 'foreign object' which has little identity, or the woman may identify with 'her' pregnancy. In the first case, she may be ambivalent about being pregnant, in the second, the pregnancy has fulfilled one of her desires. Between the 15th and 20th weeks, the first movements of the baby are felt; *'quickening' has occurred. Now the expectant mother perceives her baby as having an identity of its own, with whom she has to establish a relationship. During late pregnancy, a further change occurs, as the woman waits impatiently for the birth, but may be anxious about whether her baby will be healthy and undamaged.

These concerns during pregnancy, and the hormonal changes occurring in a pregnant woman's body, combine to affect her behaviour. Swings of mood and episodes of fatigue occur in the early months, to be replaced, as pregnancy advances, by increased feelings of passivity and dependency. Some women tend to withdraw; others express concern about the effects of their enlarging body and their altered sexual feelings on their relationship with their husband or partner. If the man is supportive, the anxiety is reduced, but some women become depressed or anxious and require additional help.

Psychoprophylaxis

Because childbirth was until recently seen as a mystery, attended by pain, and the possibility of death, it was believed that a 'conditioned reflex' developed increasing the fear of childbirth and magnified the pain of uterine contractions. Psychoprophylaxis seeks to eliminate the 'conditioned reflex' by increasing the knowledge of the woman (and her partner) of the process of childbirth, and by raising the level at which she translates uterine contractions into pain in her mind. If the woman can learn techniques to raise her pain threshold and to help herself in the stages of childbirth, it will be a less painful process.

The changes are made in two ways. First, the woman attends group discussions in which she shares experiences and attitudes towards pregnancy and labour and learns about the process of childbirth. She is also taught to perceive a uterine contraction as a signal for relaxation and controlled breathing rather than for tension or pain. Second, she is taught methods of relaxation, massage, and breathing exercises to give her a greater awareness of her body so that she can understand and work with the contractions when she starts in labour. This is learned by practising the skills she will need during childbirth together with her partner (or some other supporting person) who will be with her when she goes into labour. The results are enhanced if those who attend the woman during labour inform her of progress and encourage her to maintain the neuromuscular control she has learned.

Using psychoprophylaxis, one woman in 10 is not helped; nearly half require fewer pain-killers than expected and half require none at all.

Puberty

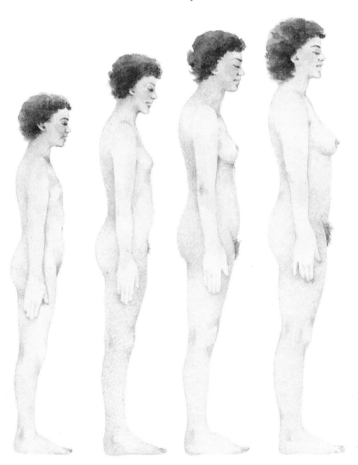

Adolescence extends from childhood to maturity and, during this time, a period of rapid change in the child's body occurs over 2 to 3 years. This is termed puberty, and its most significant mark in females is the onset of ★menstruation (menarche). Menarche occurs following a period of growth in height and weight, and seems to depend to some extent on the girl laying down a critical amount of fat in her body. The growth spurt is caused by the secretion of pituitary hormones which also stimulate the ovaries to secrete ★oestrogen. Oestrogen, in turn, stimulates the development of the girl's breasts, particularly the nipple area; enables fat to be deposited in the breast tissues so that they become rounded; leads to the growth of the internal and external genital organs and 'primes' the uterus for menstruation; enables fat to be deposited on the hips and thighs; induces the onset of menstruation. Menarche occurs on average at the age of 12½, but it is normal if it occurs in the age range 9 to 17. Menarche which occurs earlier than the age of 9 is termed ★precocious puberty, that which occurs after the age of 16 is ★delayed puberty. The physical changes of puberty are matched by psychological changes, as the girl becomes concerned about the appearance of her body and its development. Often this leads to dieting or an ★eating disorder.

Pubic lice

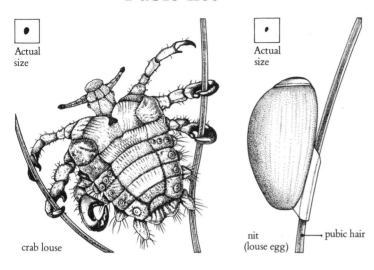

Actual size

crab louse

Actual size

nit (louse egg) → pubic hair

Pubic lice are relatives of head lice and may infest pubic hair. They are wingless insects the size of a pinhead, and are called crabs or 'crab lice' because of their appearance. Lice cannot jump and are transferred from person to person usually during sexual intercourse, when the pubic areas of both participants are in close contact. Occasionally they may be transferred from infested bedding or towels. The lice clasp pubic hair with claws on their hind feet, which makes them difficult to pick off. They feed by biting into the skin and sucking blood. This may cause itching and the infested person begins to scratch. The female louse lays about 8 eggs each day and cements them to the hairs. After a week the nits hatch and the infestation spreads. Occasionally head lice may also infest pubic hair.

Treatment of lice of any kind is to apply shampoos or lotions containing 1% gamma benzene hexachloride, or malathion 1%, which is claimed to be less irritating to the skin. While the skin is still wet the pubic area should be combed with a fine-toothed metal comb to remove the nits. This is rather time-consuming but essential, and the infested person should stand on a large piece of newspaper which can be crumpled and burned, together with the nits. After combing, the pubic area should be rinsed thoroughly. This treatment should be repeated the following day. And it may need to be repeated again.

Quickening

Between the 16th and 20th week of pregnancy, the mother feels the first movements of the fetus. The first movements are usually 'fluttering', but some women say that they feel the baby kicking from the beginning. When the mother perceives that the fetus is moving, the baby is said to have 'quickened'.

In previous centuries quickening was regarded as the first time that the fetus was 'animated' or alive, and a pregnant woman whose baby had quickened could not be hanged for murder until after the child was born. Doctors use the onset of quickening as a means of dating pregnancy.

Rape

Rape is a sexual assault, usually on a girl or a woman, in which the person is threatened or forced to have vaginal, oral, or anal intercourse against her consent. It is also a sexual assault if she is forced to masturbate the man or to be masturbated by the man. Rape may occur by force, fear, or fraud, and in some countries a husband may be held to have raped his wife. Male rapists are usually single, under the age of 30, often abuse alcohol or drugs, and in half of all cases are known to the woman. Most rapists are insecure in their relationships with other people, and obtain excitement from causing fear or pain and from their ability to humiliate the person they rape.

A woman who has been raped usually feels 'used' and dirty and some are damaged physically as well as mentally. Because of society's attitudes to human sexuality and the woman's fear of being humiliated further, many cases of rape go unreported. This is changing, and a woman who has been raped can obtain the considerable emotional support she needs from experienced counsellors, who often work from a 'Rape Crisis Centre' or similar place. The counsellors are usually women (as are the doctors) and help the woman come to terms with her pain and anger at being sexually abused, and give her the opportunity to determine what she will do. If the person who has been raped wishes to obtain redress for the assault it is important that she remembers exactly what took place, and in what sequence, so that it can be told as matter of factly as possible; that she avoids showering, washing the genitals, or changing the appearance of her clothes until she has seen a doctor; and avoids drinking any alcohol before talking to the police, as she may be accused of being drunk and willingly submitting to the rapist.

Retrolental fibroplasia

This is a condition which causes blindness in ★preterm babies who have been treated with high concentrations of oxygen over a period of time, to enable their immature lungs to take up oxygen and keep them alive. Once it was the largest single cause of blindness in Britain and the United States, but when it was realized that excessive oxygen was the cause, the amount of oxygen in the air given to a baby in an incubator was reduced and carefully monitored. As a result, retrolental fibroplasia is uncommon today.

Retroverted uterus

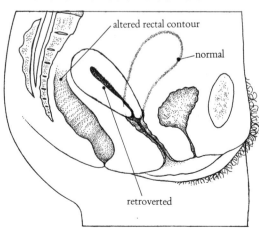

altered rectal contour

normal

retroverted

Usually the uterus lies in the woman's pelvis, angled forward (anteverted) and bent forward on itself (anteflexed). In about 10 per cent of women, the uterus is angled backward (retroverted). Provided the uterus is movable (when the woman is examined) and she does not have a ★pelvic infection or ★endometriosis, there is no cause for concern and treatment to correct the position of the uterus is unnecessary and not indicated. In past years, many gynaecological disorders were attributed to retroversion of the uterus. These included backache, sterility, pelvic pain, diminished sexual desire, failure to reach orgasm, and constipation – among others. Many operations were devised, many doctors grew richer, and many women continued to have symptoms, for none of the conditions listed is due to a retroverted uterus. Some doctors even *induced* ill health by saying that the uterus was 'twisted' (a frightening concept), which was entirely untrue as the uterus is tilted backwards, not twisted backwards.

Surgery to treat a retroverted uterus is only required if the uterus is firmly fixed by endometriosis or infection and is causing symptoms in the patient, such as painful sexual intercourse.

Rhesus iso-immune disease

Human beings can be divided into two groups by means of a blood test. One group, which has a substance called rhesus attached to their red blood cells, account for 85 per cent of the population of Europe and the United States. The second group does not have the rhesus antigen attached to their red cells and they are called Rhesus-negative (Rh-negative). Since 85 per cent of people are Rhesus-positive and 15 per cent Rhesus-negative, the odds are that in one marriage in 10 the woman will be Rh-negative and the man Rh-positive. If they decide to have a baby it may be Rh-positive or Rh-negative depending on which gene it has inherited from its father. If it is Rh-negative, no problem arises; but if it is Rh-positive, problems may occur with a later pregnancy, although the first baby will not be affected. In late pregnancy, small numbers of the baby's Rh-positive red blood cells may seep across the *placenta and enter the mother's blood stream, where they are destroyed. At delivery, however, much larger amounts of fetal blood get into the mother's blood stream. The amount may be too great to be destroyed immediately, and the surviving cells are recognized as being foreign invaders, marked as Rh-positive. The mother's defence system goes into action and special commando cells, called immuno-competent cells, manufacture a destructive substance (or antibody) which attaches itself to the foreign Rh-positive cells, coats their surface, clumps them and literally blows them apart. Once stimulated, the mother's defence system remains on the alert should any further Rh-positive cells enter her body.

The same couple decide to have a further child. Again it inherits half its genes from its father, and again it may be Rh-positive. If it is, the anti-Rh antibody, which the mother's immuno-competent cells have continued to manufacture, circulates through her blood stream, and because of its peculiar shape is able to pass through the placenta and may enter the blood stream of the fetus. This does not happen in early pregnancy, but becomes more likely as pregnancy advances. In the blood stream of the fetus, the antibody encounters the baby's Rh-positive red blood cells and coats them so that they burst. The burst red cells release a substance called bilirubin, which accumulates in the baby's blood, and some of it is excreted into the *amniotic sac in the baby's urine. As its red blood cells are destroyed, the baby becomes progressively so anaemic that it is bloated, Buddha-like, and dies; this is called hydrops fetalis. If fewer red blood cells are destroyed, the baby remains alive but is born anaemic and jaundiced from the accumulation of bilirubin in its blood.

It is now possible to prevent this occurring by testing all pregnant women in early pregnancy to determine their rhesus group. If the woman is Rh-negative and her baby at birth is found to be Rh-positive, she can be given an injection of rhesus antibody which will coat all the fetal blood cells in her circulation before they can 'sensitize' her to form her own anti-Rh antibodies. Unfortunately, if she has already become sensitized (by having had a Rh-positive baby previously), the injection is of no use. In these cases it is possible to find out firstly, if the Rh-negative mother has been stimulated to manufacture antibodies, by doing a test on her blood; and secondly, to determine how badly the baby is likely to be affected, by taking a sample of the amniotic fluid and estimating the amount of bilirubin in it. This test on the amniotic fluid is done first at about 28 weeks, and may be repeated once or twice more. The object of these tests is to find out when it is more dangerous for the baby to be inside the uterus than to be born. Once born, its damaged blood can be replaced in an 'exchange transfusion' by Rh-negative blood, which the antibodies cannot attack since the red cells have no antigen on their surface. The transfused blood keeps the baby alive while such antibodies as remain slowly decay over the following weeks. Some babies need further transfusions, but by the 6th week of life, all the antibodies transferred from the mother have decayed. Using these methods, most affected babies now survive, but a few still die in the uterus. The death of about half of these babies can be prevented by giving the baby a transfusion of Rh-negative blood. This can be carried out by means of *fetoscopy, where a fetoscope is inserted into the uterus of the mother and blood is transfused directly into a vein, or alternatively it can be done by inserting a needle through the uterus and into the baby's abdomen, under *ultrasound screening.

Rheumatism

Rheumatism is a term which includes two diseases: rheumatoid arthritis and osteoarthritis. Although different, the two diseases have similar symptoms, namely stiffness of the joints after periods of rest, which usually shows as early morning stiffness and is reduced with exercise; pain in the affected joint, which is usually described as a dull, aching sensation; and occasional swelling of the joint.

Rheumatoid arthritis affects 3 women in every 100, usually aged between 25 and 55, and in some cases there is a family history of the disease. The cause of rheumatoid arthritis is unknown, but the disease may be caused by a virus, which stimulates the body to make antibodies which damage its own tissues. Rheumatoid arthritis may affect any joint, but the joints of the hands, feet, and knees are most commonly affected, and in about 20 per cent of women small 'nodules' appear beneath the skin over the joint where it rubs repetitively against some surface.

Osteoarthritis is a disease which affects the cartilage of the joint, which swells and over the years becomes eroded by the movement of the joint. For this reason osteoarthritis is usually a disease of older people.

Both forms of arthritis seem to be increasing in frequency, perhaps as the numbers of older people increase in the community. Because of this, doctors are paying greater attention to the diseases which, although disabling, rarely cause death. In acute cases of rheumatoid arthritis, hospital treatment, often involving splinting and physiotherapy, is helpful, but most people have chronic rheumatism and need to learn methods of coping with the disease and 'tricks' which they can use to reduce the discomfort. Advice from a physiotherapist is invaluable, and exercise is beneficial. Swimming is particularly helpful as it maintains and promotes muscle tone and strength. The 'tricks' learned help the person to cope with daily living, particularly in doing the housework and preparing meals. Some people who have rheumatism become depressed and may need help in coming to terms with their disability. Much help can be obtained from friends and from voluntary agencies that are formed to help sufferers.

Drugs help many rheumatism sufferers, but they should only be taken after consultation and in accordance with a doctor's advice. It is usual to start with simple anti-inflammatory drugs, such as aspirin or one of the newer 'non-steroidal anti-inflammatory' drugs. In some cases of rheumatoid arthritis, an injection of corticosteroid into a joint may be required. Other doctors recommend gold injections or tablets of penicillamine. The latter has to be taken for several weeks before an improvement is observed. In osteoarthritis, the non-steroidal anti-inflammatory drugs help to relieve discomfort, and occasionally surgery is beneficial. The surgery may be to 'fuse' the joint or to replace the damaged portion with a plastic joint. Hip replacements have proved to give excellent results in people over the age of 50, and knee replacement is now possible but has not been performed for long enough to say how successful it will continue to be over a number of years. Surgery may also help people whose rheumatoid arthritis has led to destruction of the joint or to deformity, particularly of the wrist and ankle.

Rooming-in

In recent years increasing numbers of hospitals allow the mother to keep her baby beside her for all of the day and, generally, overnight as well. This is called 'rooming-in'. Rooming-in has several advantages. First of all, the mother and baby are treated as a 'unit', and the chance of cross-infection is eliminated. Secondly, rooming-in enables the mother to become adjusted to her baby and to interpret his needs at a time when experienced people are available to reassure her. Rooming-in is particularly appropriate if a woman chooses to breast-feed her baby, as it is known that lactation is encouraged if a woman picks up and feeds her baby when it needs to be fed. As the baby is beside his mother, she is therefore able to meet his needs when he articulates them by crying. These needs may be for food, for warmth, or for close bodily contact, all of which can readily be given if the baby and mother are together.

Rubella in pregnancy

In most Western countries, over 85 per cent of women have had an attack of rubella (German measles) before reaching the age of 16 and are therefore protected against any further infection by the rubella virus. This means that if they become pregnant their fetus is also protected.

Women who have not had rubella, or have not been immunized against the disease, may contract rubella when they are pregnant. If the infection occurs in the first 12 weeks of pregnancy, one baby in 3 will be malformed, often severely. Some babies develop cataracts, others are deaf, others have heart defects, others have poor general development or mental retardation.

These disasters can be avoided in two ways. In some countries, such as the United Kingdom and Australia, all schoolgirls aged 13 or 14 receive rubella vaccine. In others blood samples of women intending to become pregnant are checked by measuring anti-rubella antibodies to find if the woman is immune to rubella. Those with no antibodies are offered rubella vaccine, but must avoid pregnancy for 3 months.

If a woman has not been tested before she becomes pregnant, the test is usually made at the first antenatal visit. If the amount of antibody (titre) is raised, there is no need to worry or for further tests to be made. A low antibody titre level or the absence of antibodies shows that the woman may be infected if she comes into contact with rubella. If this occurs, further tests are made about three weeks after the contact, when a rise in titre indicates she has recently been infected. After full discussion the couple may decide to have the pregnancy terminated, because of the likelihood of serious malformation or illness of the fetus. Rubella vaccine is now offered to non-immune women soon after childbirth. It can be given whether the mother is breast-feeding or not.

Safe period

*Ovulation occurs 13 to 15 days (usually 14 days) before the start of the next menstrual period, and the egg (ovum) has a life-span of 2 days, unless it is fertilized by a sperm. Sperms can only fertilize an egg for about 3 days after being ejaculated. It is unlikely that pregnancy will occur if sexual intercourse is avoided for 3 days before and 3 days after ovulation. The remaining days of the menstrual cycle, excluding these six days, are therefore called the 'safe' period. Unfortunately, the duration of any woman's menstrual cycle varies, and consequently several methods have been devised in order to identify the safe period (see *Natural family planning methods).

Salpingectomy

Salpingectomy is the removal of a *Fallopian tube. The operation may be necessary if a tube has become infected, and there has been an accumulation of pus (more correctly called a pyosalpinx) or if the Fallopian tube has become swollen and filled with fluid (a hydrosalpinx). The operation may be used to treat an *ectopic pregnancy, or as a method of permanent birth control, although in such cases only a part of the tube is usually removed (this is known as *tubal ligation or sterilization).

Salpingitis

In this condition the Fallopian tubes are infected, becoming swollen, red, and tender. The infection is usually part of a *pelvic infection. It is caused by bacteria which reach the Fallopian tube following intercourse with a man infected with *gonorrhoea or *non-gonococcal urethritis, after an infected abortion, or following infection after childbirth. The treatment is to prescribe antibiotics. If treatment is not given, and occasionally when it is, the woman may be made permanently sterile.

Scabies

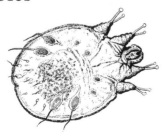

This worldwide skin disease is caused by a small mite, *Sarcoptes scabiei*, or its Norwegian cousin. The scabies mite obtains food by burrowing into the outer layers of the skin; the female also lays her eggs in the burrow which then hatch and form fresh burrows. The burrows are surrounded by an oblong area of reddened inflamed skin and are very itchy. They are usually found in the webs between the fingers, the fold of the wrists or elbows, under the breasts in women or on the buttocks. They can infest the genitals.

The saliva from the mites and their droppings are irritating to the skin and cause the intense itch, especially when the person is warm, or in bed. The person scratches, which makes the spots bleed and become infected. The Norwegian version is more severe and often the spots become covered with a crust of pus. As the rash can be mistaken for a syphilitic rash, a blood test should be made if a sexually active adult develops scabies. Treatment is to have a bath and scrub the whole body (except the face and neck) gently with a soft brush and then apply a lotion of benzyl benzoate or 1% gamma benzene hexachloride. The treatment is repeated for 3 days and clothes should be laundered each day. At the end of the treatment all underclothes, pillows, and sheets should be laundered and ironed.

Scabies is highly contagious, the mite being transferred by skin contact (not be genital contact), so other members of the infected person's family should be examined.

Semen analysis

About one couple in 7 find that they are unable to conceive a child, in spite of trying for one year. In one-third of these couples, the defect seems to be in the quality or quantity of the semen ejaculated by the man. For this reason when infertility is investigated, a specimen of semen is examined in a laboratory. The man produces the specimen by masturbating, or by being stimulated to orgasm by his partner, or by having sexual intercourse and withdrawing just before he ejaculates. In each case the semen is ejaculated into a dry, warmed glass or plastic container (a small jam jar is excellent, although plastic is less likely to cool the sperm). Most men prefer to provide the specimen at home. A note is made of the time at which the specimen is produced, and it must be taken to the laboratory within 2 hours. In the laboratory the volume is measured, and the number of *spermatozoa are counted under a microscope. Also counted is the number of

spermatozoa which are still active and the percentage of spermatozoa with abnormally shaped heads or bodies.

As a guide, the man is fertile if the following are found:

Volume : more than 2 ml
Count : more than 20 million
per ml
'Normally shaped
sperm' : more than 60 per cent
Mortality at 4 hours : 40 per cent

If the examination indicates that the man has less than 20 million spermatozoa per ml of semen, the test is repeated twice, at about a week's interval, before any evaluation is made. If the sperm count is less than 5 million per ml, blood tests to measure certain hormones are made, so that the doctor can decide whether any treatment is available which may improve the man's sperm count and his chance of fertilizing his partner.

Sex determination

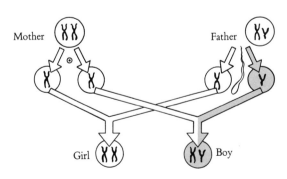

Mother   Father

Girl   Boy

The sex of the baby is determined by the combination of the X chromosomes of the mother with either the X or the Y contained in the father's sperm. Boys will be XY and girls XX

The human body is made up of millions of cells. Each cell contains in its nucleus 46 *chromosomes, with two notable exceptions, the spermatozoa in men and the egg cells (ova) in women. Forty-four of the chromosomes in the cells are body chromosomes and 2 are sex chromosomes. There are two kinds of sex chromosomes, called X and Y because of their shape. A woman's body cells contain 44 body chromosomes and 2 X chromosomes. This is written as 46XX. A man's body cells contain 44 body chromosomes, one X chromosome, and one Y chromosome, written 46XY.

Each egg contains half the number of chromosomes found in body cells, that is, 22 body chromosomes plus one X chromosome. Spermatozoa are of two chromosomal types: they may contain 22 body chromosomes plus one X chromosome or 22 body chromosomes plus one Y chromosome.

If a sperm carrying an X chromosome fertilizes the egg, the new individual's cells will have a complement of 46XX and the person will be female. If a sperm carrying a Y chromosome fertilizes an egg, the new individual's cells will have a complement of 46XY, and the person will be male.

For as long as history has been recorded, couples have wanted to be able to choose the sex of their child. It is known that an infant's sex is determined by the father's spermatozoa. Since the same numbers of X and Y spermatozoa are found in the semen, chance determines the sex of the child. Reports have recently been published which suggest that more girls than boys are produced if intercourse takes place 2 or 3 days before *ovulation and the couple then abstain from sex; and that more boys than girls are produced if intercourse is avoided until after ovulation and the woman douches with an alkaline vaginal solution before intercourse. These reports are contradicted by other reports which show exactly the opposite. At present – and perhaps for a long time to come – a couple cannot choose the sex of their baby. Chance determines it.

Sex education

The need for education in human sexuality (including relationships, contraception, and sexually transmitted diseases) during childhood and adolescence continues to arouse strong emotions. There is also fierce debate about who should provide such education. Some groups believe sex education to be the sole responsibility of the parents. Others point out that many parents are relatively uninformed about sexuality or perpetuate myths, and that sex education in such instances will be either minimal or misleading. Most carefully conducted investigations, particularly when children's views are taken into account, suggest that sex education should begin in the home, but should be supplemented by instruction at school. The studies show that a large gap exists between what children want to know and what they have been told. It has also been shown that most children believe that the information they received was provided too late.

Children from the age of 8 onwards are capable of understanding quite complex biological concepts, provided that the person giving the information does so in a relaxed and natural way and uses appropriate vocabulary. In the absence of this approach, children acquire their own explanation for sexual processes, usually in the form of myths, from their peers. They also acquire information about sexuality from the magazines, books and newspapers they read and the television programmes and films they see. This material is frequently presented in a sensational manner.

The consensus of informed opinion is that parents may themselves need assistance in acquiring knowledge about human sexuality so that they can transmit information to their children; and by their actions can provide models of appropriate sexual behaviour. In addition, a systematic programme of sexual education needs to be provided at school. This programme should start in primary school and continue into secondary school.

The purpose of the programme is not merely to provide sufficient sexual knowledge but to be the basis for subsequent sexual development. Such a programme might include the following:

1 It should describe the physical, mental, and emotional changes which occur during *puberty to girls and boys. This information must include details of *genital anatomy and its variations, and discussions to reduce anxiety about *menstruation, *masturbation, *petting, wet dreams, and sexual arousal.

2 It should explain about conception, pregnancy, childbirth, and parenthood. It should also stress the obligations and responsibilities of the couple to each other and to their child.

3 It should give accurate information about *contraception and birth control. This should be provided initially before the child reaches puberty and should be reinforced and expanded during later school years, when many students are already exploring their own sexuality and experimenting and when advice is most necessary.

4 It should provide clear information about ★sexually transmitted diseases and the dangers involved.

5 It should encourage students to accept people whose sexual practices are discordant with their own.

6 Most importantly, it should provide the basis for sexual responsibility in which the obligations of one human to another are emphasized, the conditions which encourage sexual exploitation are discussed, and sexual mythology is replaced by sexual knowledge.

Sex selection

It is known that if a spermatozoon carrying an X chromosome fertilizes an egg, the new individual will be female; while if the egg is fertilized by a spermatozoon carrying a Y chromosome, the new individual will be male. If it were possible to separate all the X-carrying spermatozoa from all the Y-carrying spermatozoa, it would be possible for parents to choose the sex of the child. This is not possible. Doctors have suggested methods of doing this, but none has proved better than chance, in spite of claims by doctors and parents who achieved the sex they desired. Perhaps in the future techniques will be developed to allow sex selection for use in sex-linked congenital diseases.

Sexual desire

Sexual desire (libido) is the psychological urge by which people are sexually attracted to each other and become sexually aroused. Why one person should be attracted sexually to another but ignore the third, is not clear. One suggestion is that each person develops her or his unique sexual 'scenario', starting in childhood. In this scenario, the person is the hero, and the 'script' is modified repeatedly as new experiences are absorbed. The 'writer' creates and identifies the sort of person who arouses her sexually and towards whom she feels sexual desire. When she meets that person she desires to make closer contact.

This contact may confirm the desire, or the behaviour and attitudes of the other person may extinguish it. If sexual desire is stimulated, the contact will become even closer, and the senses of sight, sound, smell, and touch will transmit impulses to the brain, which will be converted into the feeling of sexual arousal; or the reverse may occur, and the couple will separate. Libido is the term applied to sexual desire and to the beginning of sexual arousal. A person with a high libido is easily aroused, a person who has a low libido may not feel much sexual desire and is not easily aroused.

Sexual intercourse

It is a comment on society's inhibitions that there is no 'polite' word to describe a universal activity. The only single words are in Latin or are considered vulgar or obscene. Sexual intercourse means that the penis penetrates the vagina and thrusting movements take place. Sexual intercourse should be a shared pleasure in which each partner has found out what gives the other the most enjoyment, and which activities are found unpleasant by the other person. Sexual intercourse is most enjoyable when a compromise is reached and both partners enjoy the act. The most common position for sexual intercourse is with the man on top of the woman (the 'missionary' position); but any position which produces pleasure for both partners is normal. Increasingly, younger unmarried people are sexually active, so that in most Western countries 75 per cent of men and 70 per cent of women have had sexual intercourse by the age of 19.

Sexual pleasuring

Sexual pleasuring is the process of stimulation of the erogenous parts of the body which leads to sexual arousal. In the past it was called foreplay, implying that all sexual stimulation was expected to end with the man inserting his penis into the woman's vagina. This concept is now outdated, as other ways to reach orgasm are accepted, and sexual pleasuring itself is recognized as a complete form of love-making. Sexual pleasuring implies that each partner finds out from the other what particular methods are sexually stimulating (such as massage, kissing, *fellatio, *cunnilingus, and so on), and which parts of their body are the most erogenous. The couple may always use the same method of pleasuring, or may add variety and play sexual games with each other. The ways in which people pleasure each other sexually are many and varied: all are acceptable provided each partner agrees beforehand, and if a method is found unpleasant it is stopped.

Sexual problems

In the past, sexual problems were separated from problems in a relationship. It is now realized that sexual problems may arise because of a poor relationship between the partners, or they may occur because of fear of sexuality resulting from inhibited attitudes to sex. Many women have sexual or relationship problems but accept them. It is only when the woman is able to talk about her problem to her partner or when she seeks professional help that it is realized that she has a problem. There are three main problems of a relationship/sexual nature. These are inhibition of sexual desire; painful intercourse (dyspareunia and vaginismus); and failure to achieve orgasm (anorgasmia).

A woman who has *inhibited sexual desire* does not feel sexually attracted to another person, and if a person attempts to excite her sexually by sex play, she finds the experience distasteful. Inhibited sexual desire only becomes a problem if a woman is placed in a situation where she is expected to respond sexually, and fails to do so. She may avoid such situations, and may never desire sexual pleasure, or she may obtain this herself by masturbating.

Painful intercourse (dyspareunia) may be caused by vaginal infections, pelvic disease, or local conditions in the woman's genitals; or it may have a psychological origin. The condition should only be considered to be of psychological origin when physical causes have been excluded. The woman may feel pain when her partner tries to insert his penis, or when he is deep inside her, and thrusts. In extreme cases, the woman feels unable to permit her partner to insert his penis, clamping her legs together and contracting the muscles around her vaginal opening. This condition is called *vaginismus* (which means vaginal spasm). She may enjoy touching, kissing, having her breasts fondled, but cannot permit her partner to touch her genital area. If a woman seeks treatment for dyspareunia, the physical causes are first eliminated or treated. Then the woman is invited to talk with a trained therapist who tries to help her see why she fears intercourse, and to suggest ways by which she can lose the fear. Many women who complain of vaginismus have no knowledge of their *genital anatomy. The therapist lets the woman look at her external genitals in a mirror and explains the anatomy. The woman is then invited to try and insert her own finger into her vagina, or to permit the doctor to introduce a finger. The woman learns that this procedure is not painful, and quite quickly is able to introduce two and then three fingers, or allow a vaginal *speculum to be introduced. In these ways she learns that it will not be painful for her to accept her partner's penis.

Failure to achieve orgasm (anorgasmia) Studies have shown that only about 50 per cent of women reach orgasm during sexual intercourse, but that over 90 per cent of women can reach orgasm if the clitoral area is stimulated by finger, her partner's tongue, or if she uses a *vibrator. The idea that a woman must reach orgasm during every episode of sexual intercourse and, preferably, simultaneously with her partner is unrealistic. Treatment of anorgasmia begins when her therapist helps her to express her feelings about sex, and to

learn about her genital anatomy. Her feelings about masturbation are explored and, if she feels comfortable, she learns how to masturbate using a vibrator or her finger. She may want her partner to be involved. This approach is often beneficial, as it encourages communication between them when she can learn about her body as they caress each other and can tell her partner what gives her pleasure and what does not. She finds that she is able to have an enjoyable orgasm with her partner's help and they both learn her pattern of *sexual response, so that they can adjust their sex play accordingly to give it maximum expression.

Sexual response in women

For descriptive purposes, the human sexual response can be divided into five phases, although the distinction between the phases is often blurred. These phases are sexual desire; sexual arousal or excitement; sexual plateau; orgasm; sexual resolution.

Sexual desire begins when a person sees another to whom she is attracted. Why one person is attracted to another but not to a third is not understood, but it may be because of experiences, observation, and fantasy which creates in the woman's mind an image of a person to whom she could be attracted. Sexual desire is increased if contact with the other person, when they meet, talk, look, and perhaps touch each other, confirms the attraction. In the event of sexual desire and attraction leading to a relationship, the subsequent phase of the human sexual response is likely to occur.

Sexual arousal or excitement is initiated more by body contact than by sight or sound. During this phase, the blood vessels supplying the genital area and the nipples dilate, so that the amount of blood in these tissues increases. The clitoris increases in size, mainly in width, and the 'lips' around the vaginal entrance become softer and thicker as they become congested with blood, forming soft swellings. These changes vary in degree from woman to woman.

At the same time, fluid enters the pelvic tissues, the vagina becomes softer, and some

of the fluid seeps through the layers of tiny cells which make up the vaginal wall, so that it becomes lubricated. Two small organs (Bartholin's glands) which lie near the opening of the vagina also secrete fluid, so that both the vagina and its entrance become moist and slippery. If the man attempts to introduce his penis before the fluid has been secreted and the area has become lubricated, intercourse may be painful. Simultaneously, the tissues surrounding the lower third of the woman's vagina become swollen with blood, so that soft, warm 'cushions' form which will caress the man's penis as it enters the vagina. The woman's nipples become erect and the surrounding areola becomes swollen.

Sexual plateau This stage is reached when sexual excitement is intense, and it is a continuation of the excitement phase. The woman's heart rate increases, her blood pressure rises, and a reddish rash may appear on the skin of her abdomen or breasts. The vagina lengthens and the clitoris seems to disappear under its hood. The congestion of the pelvic tissues is at its maximum at this time and will remain until orgasm has occurred (this is why this phase is called the 'plateau' stage).

Orgasm Descriptions given by women suggest that an orgasm is a feeling of intense pleasure which is the peak of sexual arousal. Initially, the feeling is usually located deep in

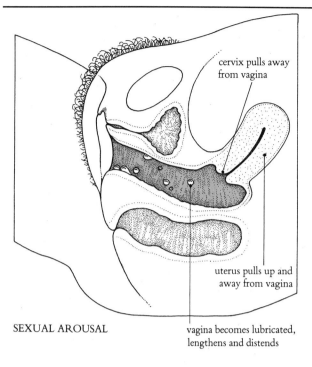

cervix pulls away
from vagina

uterus pulls up and
away from vagina

SEXUAL AROUSAL

vagina becomes lubricated,
lengthens and distends

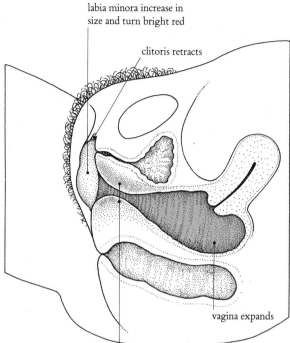

labia minora increase in
size and turn bright red

clitoris retracts

vagina expands

PLATEAU STAGE

swelling of tissues to produce cushions;
vaginal entrance contracts to produce
a grasping effect

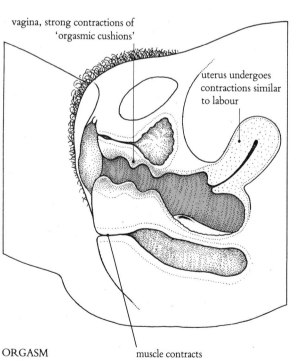

vagina, strong contractions of
'orgasmic cushions'

uterus undergoes
contractions similar
to labour

ORGASM

muscle contracts

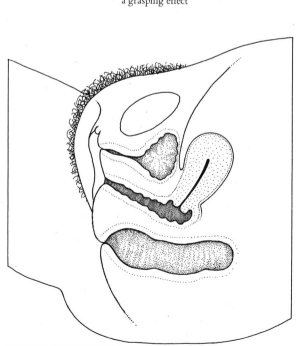

SEXUAL RESOLUTION – return to non-aroused state

the pelvis, but later it spreads over the whole body. During the orgasm the woman's feelings are concentrated on the sensations, largely to the exclusion of anything else. It begins with moments of stillness which are followed by uncontrollable muscle movements, a general tingling, a floating feeling, warmth, well-being, a release of mental tension, and exhilaration.

An orgasm is due to a reflex. Stimulation of the clitoral area, either directly when a woman masturbates or is caressed, or indirectly by the movement of the man's penis as he thrusts in her vagina, sends a message to her spinal cord. In the spinal cord, the reflex occurs and the message is relayed to the nerves which control the muscles of the pelvis. But whether the message is relayed at all, is increased in its intensity, or is inhibited, depends on the degree of control by her brain over the reflex. A woman who has no inhibitions about sex will probably enhance the strength of the message and will have an orgasm. If she has inhibitions or does not like the feeling that the man is 'using' her, she may fail to have an orgasm during intercourse, although she can reach an orgasm by fantasizing when she masturbates.

A woman's orgasm may be associated with the same thrusting movements of the thigh and pelvic muscles as those of a man, but some women remain still during the orgasm. A woman's orgasm only differs from a man's by the absence of ejaculation.

In most orgasms, the 'trigger' which starts the orgasm reflex is the stimulated clitoris, although additional messages may come from stimulation of the vagina. In all people, an orgasm is expressed by contractions of the deep pelvic muscles including those of the vagina in women and is felt as pleasure by a special area of the brain. Until recently, many women believed that men 'gave' them orgasms and if a woman failed to have an orgasm during intercourse she was lacking in femininity and would make the man feel sexually inadequate. Because of this many women 'faked' orgasms so that the man would not feel inadequate or she unfeminine. With a more open approach to women's sexuality, it is now known that women who fail to reach orgasm during intercourse are not deficient in sexual drive, and that to 'fake' an orgasm is folly.

About one-third of women reach an orgasm with every, or nearly every, episode of sexual intercourse, and one woman in every 3 in this group is able to have multiple orgasms. More than 50 per cent of women occasionally reach a climax during sexual intercourse and consistently do so if the clitoris is stimulated with the man's finger or his tongue before or after he has had an orgasm, or if the woman masturbates. Only about 10 per cent of women reach an orgasm very occasionally or never.

Sexual resolution In both sexes, the convulsive muscle contractions and the deep pleasure of orgasm are followed by relaxation. But in contrast to a man's penis, the clitoris is usually not tender and some women can have several orgasms with a minimal interval between each one. In the first five to ten minutes of the resolution phase the tissues of the vagina and the vulva lose the fluid which had seeped into them. The congestion diminishes and the swelling of the tissues disappears as they return to the non-aroused state.

Sexuality, double standard

The sexual double standard implies that women should remain virgins until marriage and faithful thereafter, but men may engage in sex before marriage and to a lesser extent after marriage. The concept developed when it was assumed that men had a far stronger sexual urge than women, and when it was essential that a man be sure that any child of a union was his. Even in the relatively permissive sexual climate current in Western society, the sexual double standard continues to be accepted by many people.

Sexuality in pregnancy and after childbirth

The psychological, physical, and hormonal changes of pregnancy have a profound effect on a woman's sexuality. In general, as pregnancy advances, women have a reduced desire for sex and respond less. The reduction in sexuality is due to a variety of causes. First, some women are afraid that sexual intercourse will bring on labour prematurely or may hurt the baby. Second, in late pregnancy sexual intercourse, in the traditional man-on-top position, may be uncomfortable. Third, some women see themselves as unattractive and awkward, and are concerned that their partner may see them in this way. Fourth, some doctors still prohibit sexual intercourse in the last 6 to 4 weeks of pregnancy. They do this because they believe that sexual intercourse may initiate childbirth by causing uterine contractions, or may lead to infection of the *amniotic fluid and the fetus. The evidence supporting these two beliefs is dubious. Fifth, some women should avoid sexual intercourse in late pregnancy. These include women who have an *incompetent cervix or ruptured membranes; or vaginal bleeding in late pregnancy. Apart from these three groups of women, a couple may have sexual intercourse throughout pregnancy provided the woman wants this form of sexual enjoyment and finds it comfortable.

In the first 30 weeks of pregnancy the couple may prefer the traditional man-on-top position during sexual intercourse, though after this time the position becomes uncomfortable for the woman. She may then prefer rear entry into the vagina, or the straight sideways position. If the woman finds that sexual intercourse is uncomfortable whatever position is adopted, she may prefer to be stimulated by oral or digital manipulation of her clitoral area. She may pleasure her partner by stimulating his penis with her fingers or mouth. Incidentally, swallowing spermatozoa does not lead to increased uterine activity.

After childbirth, a woman often has a reduced sexual desire and responds more slowly. Vaginal lubrication tends to be less, at least in the first two or three months. *Sexual pleasuring by cuddling, caressing, and fondling can be resumed soon after childbirth if the couple desire it. Sexual intercourse may be resumed when the woman is ready and it causes no pain. About 70 per cent of women have an *episiotomy during childbirth and in about one-fifth of cases healing is slow, so that sexual intercourse has to be avoided or is painful for several weeks or months. If this occurs, a doctor should be consulted.

The changes in sexual desire, responsiveness, and arousal (including vaginal lubrication) which occur during pregnancy and continue after the birth can affect the couple's relationship. Many of the adverse changes can be minimized if the woman's partner is aware of them and helps her to respond.

Sexually transmitted diseases

Diseases which are mainly transmitted from person to person by close sexual contact are called sexually transmitted diseases (or STDs). The sexual contact may be by *sexual intercourse, *oral sex, or *anal intercourse. The diseases, which are mentioned elsewhere in this book, include (in order of prevalence in the community) genital herpes, non-gonococcal urethritis, genital warts, gonorrhoea, syphilis, and chancroid. Many authorities also include trichomonad and candida infections, hepatitis B, and scabies.

The greater sexual freedom in Western countries in recent years has led to an increase in sexually transmitted diseases, mainly of genital herpes, non-gonococcal urethritis, and genital warts. Gonorrhoea has increased in frequency to a lesser extent, while the prevalence of syphilis seems to be on the decline.

Sheehan's syndrome
'Show'
Sims position
Skin care, dry skin

Sheehan's syndrome

In a few women who have a severe haemorrhage during pregnancy or after childbirth, with marked shock, the blood supply to the pituitary gland is severely reduced and clots may obliterate the main vessels. Because of the lack of blood, up to three-quarters of the cells which make up the pituitary gland die. As a result they are unable to secrete sufficient quantities of the pituitary hormones to keep the woman healthy, and she becomes ill. She may become lethargic and weak from a lack of the adrenal cortical and thyroid stimulating hormones; she may feel the cold excessively and may lose her appetite; *lactation will not take place, because insufficient *prolactin is produced; her menstrual periods do not return; her vagina becomes dry and her uterus shrinks in size because her pituitary gland no longer secretes the gonadotrophic hormones which stimulate her ovaries to produce *oestrogen and *progesterone, and the levels of these hormones fall; she loses her body hair; she may become thirsty and pass large quantities of urine. If untreated she may die, but given appropriate hormones by mouth or by injection, she can live a normal life. Sheehan's syndrome, as the condition is called, is increasingly rare in present times, because women who suffer from a haemorrhage are usually given adequate blood transfusions. But the condition does still occur occasionally.

'Show'

In pregnancy the cervix is 'blocked' by a plug of mucus. When labour is imminent, the cervix begins to dilate, which may cause some minor bleeding, and the mucus plug is expelled. This leads to a discharge of blood-tinged mucus from the woman's vagina. It is a 'show' that labour is about to start; and usually it does within a few hours or a few days. A show is a reasonably dependable sign of the approach of labour. If the amount of blood exceeds a few drops, the woman should report to her doctor immediately as it is possible that this may indicate an abnormal condition.

Sims position

Women often find vaginal examinations both uncomfortable and, occasionally, frightening. Usually the woman lies on her back with her legs drawn up and parted. In the United States, the woman's legs are placed in supports and her body is hidden by a drape, which can make the procedure intimidating. A few doctors ask the woman to lie on her left side, with her bottom on the edge of the examination couch and her right leg drawn up. This is the Sims position, which is named after an American gynaecologist Marion Sims, who practised in New York in the late nineteenth century.

Skin care, dry skin

Most women believe that dry or flaky skin is a condition which requires attention, or wrinkles will develop. Dry skin occurs more commonly in dry climates or among women who work for long hours in places which are air-conditioned in both summer and winter. Dry skin becomes increasingly common with age.

Cosmetic manufacturers offer a large and bewildering range of lotions and creams which moisten the skin, reducing the dry feeling, and perhaps delay the formation of wrinkles. The cost of the moisturizers varies enormously, as does their effectiveness. In the opinion of the user, this ranges from 'well above average to well below average', according to a survey of 72 products made by the Australian Consumers' Association (ACA).

The conclusion of the survey was that moisturizers do help dry skin, but that the effectiveness of the moisturizer bears no relationship to its cost: a cheap moisturizer headed the list. Nor was there any relationship between the effectiveness of the product, the user's age, the climatic conditions, or the user's skin type. This means that you waste money if you buy a moisturizer which is especially expensive, or said to be for either young or 'mature' skin, or for special weathers and seasons, or especially for 'combination' skin, according to the ACA. Nor are night creams any more effective than other moisturizers.

An effective moisturizer used night and morning after thorough cleansing of the face improves the condition of the skin for about six weeks and then maintains its condition. The ACA offers a do-it-yourself moisturizer which proved as effective as any of the commercial products. It found that Sorbolene with glycerine (and perfume if you desire) is as effective as any of the commercial preparations and is considerably cheaper. Sorbolene (cetomacrogol cream) is a basic non-prescription skin cream which many dermatologists recommend to patients who are allergic to perfume. Basically it consists of 10% liquid paraffin, 10% white soft paraffin, 5% propylene glycerol (a moistener), 15% of a non-ionic emulsifier, and 0.1% preservative made up in water.

Sorbolene with 10% added glycerine makes a pleasant hand lotion; and it is recommended by ACA as a moisturizer, when made up in the following way. 'The basic method is simple. Place the Sorbolene containing 10% added glycerine (and benzoic acid dissolved in alcohol, only if required) in a bowl, and add 100 ml of hot water (use distilled water if you wish). Beat with an old-fashioned egg-beater (we found this better than a processor). Then add the rest of the hot water and beat again. Leave to cool, and if required, beat in the perfume essence.'

Store the moisturizer in screw-top containers in the fridge, removing small quantities when you need them. An alternative is to add benzoic acid dissolved in alcohol (which your pharmacist will have to make) as a preservative. If boiled or distilled water is used to make the lotion, the chance of contamination by bacteria is reduced.

ACA offers the following recipes:

For a light lotion (the top-ranking test product)
    100 g Sorbolene (with 10%
       glycerine)
    500 ml of hot water
    (0.6 g benzoic acid if required)
    1.5 to 2.0 ml of perfume essence (if
       required)

For a heavy lotion/light cream
    100 g Sorbolene (with 10%
       glycerine)
    300 ml of hot water
    (0.4 g benzoic acid if required)
    1.5 to 2.0 ml perfume essence (if
       required)

For a mousse-type cream
    100 g Sorbolene (with 10%
       glycerine)
    150 ml of hot water
    (0.25 g benzoic acid if required)
    1.5 to 2.0 ml perfume essence (if
       required)

For a heavier cream
    100 g Sorbolene (with 10%
       glycerine)
    100 ml of hot water
    (0.2 g benzoic acid if required)
    1.5 to 2.0 ml perfume essence (if
       required)

Other cosmetic manufacturers offer women ★skin 'foods', although there is no evidence that these provide any nourishment for the cells which make up the skin. As with other body cells, the epidermis is nourished by the blood which circulates in the tissues below it. A few manufacturers offer skin cosmetics which contain ★oestrogen. The advertising which accompanies these products suggests that older women require oestrogen to keep their skin 'young'. This type of advertising is deceptive, as oestrogen does not prevent ageing. If lotions or creams containing oestrogen are used, a small amount of

Skin care, dry skin
Skin 'foods'
Small-for-dates babies

fluid is retained in, and between, the cells of the epidermis, which may make the wrinkles less apparent. Women should also be aware that oestrogen is absorbed through the skin and may have other effects on the body (see ★Hormone replacement therapy).

Skin 'foods'

Large numbers of women, persuaded by skilled advertising, purchase creams, lotions, skin tonics, and hormone preparations to delay the ★wrinkles and other signs of the ageing process in the skin. The products are lavishly launched, superbly packaged, seductively perfumed, and often very expensive. Do they do what they purport to do, namely delay the inevitable changes which occur in the skin as a woman ages? The answer is that they do not. The best way to keep the skin in good condition is by cleaning it regularly using soap and water, and drying it carefully. There is no cosmetic which will keep your skin youthful if your genetic inheritance decrees that it ages quickly. You may abuse your skin in youth, by excessive sunbathing, which will hurry the process of ageing (and may also cause skin cancer), but it is unlikely that the moisturizing creams which are purchased to limit the effects of that abuse are of any more benefit than the use of a cheap vaseline or lanolin product. This will help the skin look smooth and soft, and is just as effective as a more expensive moisturizer.

If you feel warm, loved, superior, and good when you buy expensive skin products, by all means do so. The product will do no harm, except to your pocket, and will do as much good as a cheaper product you can buy from any chemist.

Small-for-dates babies

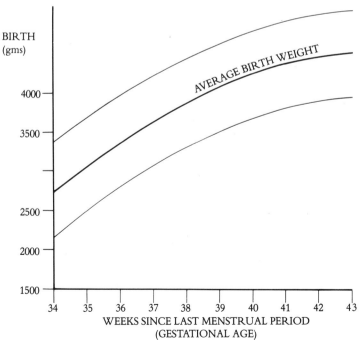

This term refers to a baby whose weight is below that expected for the period of the pregnancy. Some small-for-dates babies are also born preterm; others are born after the 37th week of pregnancy, but weigh less than expected for the period of the pregnancy. The baby is small-for-dates because he has been chronically under-nourished while growing in his mother's uterus or, to put it another way, the baby's growth is retarded. Intrauterine growth retardation occurs if the mother has conditions such as ★pre-eclampsia or chronic illness, if the baby has a ★congenital malformation or if he has been infected while he was growing. In many cases, no reason for the failure of the baby to grow is found. Small-for-dates babies require additional care and should usually be admitted to an Intensive Neonatal Care Unit (see ★Preterm birth).

The majority of babies' birth weights lie between the upper and lower line. A baby born with a birth weight below the bottom line is said to be small for dates

Smoking

Smoking is a health hazard which increases the risk of lung cancer and heart disease threefold or more. However, the habit is widespread and most smokers do not believe that they will be affected. Women who are pregnant should try to stop smoking or to reduce the number of cigarettes they smoke. This is because women who smoke (especially those smoking more than 20 cigarettes a day) are more likely to abort and to have a baby which weighs less at birth than the baby of a non-smoker and runs a greater risk of dying in the *perinatal period. It has also been found that children from households where one or both parents smoke suffer more from respiratory illnesses (such as bronchitis) than children who come from non-smoking households.

Speculum, vaginal

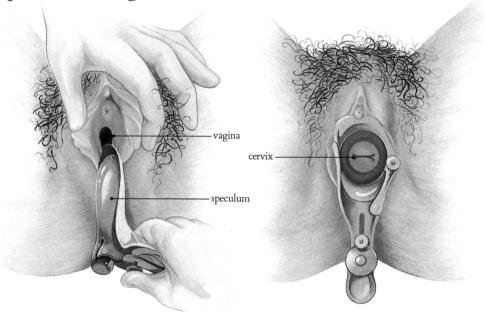

The vaginal speculum is an instrument made of metal or plastic, which is inserted into a woman's vagina so that its wall can be examined and the cervix inspected. It is also used when a swab is taken from the vagina or a *cervical smear is made. Before the speculum is inserted, a woman should ask to be shown the instrument so that she knows what is being put inside her body, and should insist that the speculum is warmed. The usual speculum is shaped like a duck's bill and once introduced is opened to expose the cervix. This places pressure on the bladder and bowel causing discomfort rather than pain. This is reduced if the woman relaxes and the doctor explains what he is doing.

Spermatozoa

The male sex cells, the spermatozoa (sperms), are produced in the man's testes at a rate of about 50000 a minute. They then spend up to 80 days in the testis or the tube (the vas deferens) which connects the testis to the prostate gland and the penis. Each spermatozoon has a head, a middle piece, and a long tail which helps it move through the woman's uterus and into her Fallopian tubes after ejaculation. When a man ejaculates, he ejects over 300 million sperms and about 3 ml of secretions, which make up over 90 per cent of the ejaculate. The secretions are of great importance, as it is these which provide nourishment for the spermatozoa waiting to be ejaculated.

Stillbirth

A baby which dies in the uterus and is born dead is called a stillbirth. Stillbirth is an old term and, until recently, in Britain only referred to a baby born from a pregnancy which had lasted 28 weeks and to a baby which weighed 1000 g or more. Today, in many countries, the term stillbirth has been replaced by the term late fetal death. Dead-born babies weighing between 500 and 1000 g are referred to as intermediate fetal deaths, and those weighing less than 500 g as early fetal deaths or abortions.

Suction curette

The suction curette (or vacuum aspirator) is used in preference to a metal curette for *menstrual regulation, inducing an *abortion, and for treating some forms of *trophoblastic disease. It consists of a plastic tube (made in sizes from 4 to 12 mm in diameter) which is connected to a container and a small pump which creates a negative pressure. The curette has an angled tip and usually two side holes. It is introduced through the cervix into the uterus, the negative pressure is created, and the contents of the uterus are sucked through the tube as the curette gently 'scrapes' the lining of the uterus. Compared with a metal curette there is less loss of blood and the suction curette is less likely to damage the uterus. The operation of suction curettage can be done either under local anaesthesia (an injection is given into the cervix) or under general anaesthesia.

Syphilis

Syphilis is a sexually transmitted disease caused by a microscopic, corkscrew-shaped organism called *Treponema pallidum*. The organism usually obtains entry to the woman's body through tiny abrasions in the skin of her labia or through her cervix. Once within her body the bacteria multiply rapidly, doubling every 30 hours. After 20 to 30 days (occasionally longer) a small sore appears on the woman's vulva and oozes serum. At this stage the sore, called a *chancre, is highly infectious. In 3 to 8 weeks the ulcer heals, leaving a scar. If syphilis is not diagnosed and treated at this stage, a secondary pale pink rash appears on the skin 6 to 8 weeks later. The spots spread over the body, then turn into pimples and sometimes into pustules, and persist for about 6 weeks when they fade. The third stage of syphilis occurs some 2 to 20 years later, when the disease either causes painful skin ulcers, heart damage, or mental decay.

The serious effects of untreated syphilis can be avoided if a woman who develops a sore with hard edges on her vulva, or a persistent rose pink rash on her body, sees a doctor. He will take a blood sample and have it tested for syphilis. If syphilis is present, it can be treated effectively with antibiotics. All pregnant women should also be tested for syphilis (the VDRL test), as undiagnosed and untreated syphilis can infect the unborn baby. This can produce specific congenital abnormalities in the newborn baby.

T

Tall girls

Some girls grow excessively tall during the spurt of growth which precedes *puberty and become much taller than other girls of the same age group. This can be psychologically disturbing. In most cases, examination shows the girl to be normal in every respect but that of height. Counselling and discussion between the girl and a health professional are important in helping her adjust to her height. But if the girl continues to feel that she is a 'freak' after counselling two treatments are available. If the girl's 'bone age' is less than 13, the hormone *oestrogen given by mouth will effectively stop her growing. Unfortunately, side-effects may occur, and the girl may choose to wait until her final height is reached (at about the age of 16). If she is still distressed by her height, surgery can be undertaken to shorten the length of her leg bones.

Teratogens

These are drugs which, if taken during the first 8 weeks or so of pregnancy, may lead to the baby being malformed. The most notorious teratogen is thalidomide. Other teratogens are cytotoxic (anti-cancer) drugs, androgenic steroids (which were formerly used to treat threatened *abortion), and corticosteroids given in large doses. From time to time reports are made, without proper study, which implicate other drugs, but in every case further research has shown that the drug was not the cause of the malformation. However, pregnant women should avoid all drugs unless they are specifically indicated and prescribed by a doctor. (See also *Drugs in pregnancy.)

Testicular feminization

She looks exactly like any other women: she has female breasts and fat distribution but she has little or no hair on her pubis and in her armpits and she does not menstruate. Her vagina ends as a short 'blind' pouch, she has no uterus. In place of ovaries she has testes. She is a male. More accurately, she has the chromosomes of a male (*karyotype) but looks and behaves as a woman. The condition is called androgenic insensitivity or testicular feminization and is due to the fact that the cells of her body lack any receptors for the male hormone testosterone, so that the body develops as a female, although testosterone is the main sex hormone circulating in the blood.

Thalassaemia

Between 5 and 10 per cent of Mediterranean people, and a smaller percentage in Asia and Africa, are affected by a form of anaemia called thalassaemia, also known as Mediterranean anaemia, which is due to the inheritance of an abnormal gene. In mild forms of the disease, the person is unaware that he or she is anaemic, until tests reveal the condition. In severe forms, the liver and spleen become enlarged, the bones may become mis-shapen, and the person requires repeated blood transfusions in order to survive; most die under the age of 20. There is no cure for the disease. The severe form occurs if both parents have the disease, though only a few of their children will inherit severe thalassaemia. The disease can now be detected before birth by testing blood from both parents, and if both are found to carry the abnormal gene, blood is taken from the fetus by introducing a needle into the uterus when the mother is about 18 weeks pregnant. If the test shows that the fetus has severe thalassaemia, termination of pregnancy can be offered. One baby in 4 will be severely affected.

Third-day blues

A number of women become temporarily depressed between the third and fifth day after childbirth. The cause of the depression has not been established. Speculation about its cause includes hormonal imbalance (although none has been identified), reaction to the excitement of childbirth, and uncertainty in the mother about her ability to care for her dependent child. Another factor in modern Western culture may be the expectation that a mother will immediately love her baby, when, in reality, *mother love is a learned behaviour. The condition, known as third-day blues, leads to bursts of crying, irritability, and in some cases general depression. It is best handled if one of the medical or nursing staff talks to the woman and explains what is happening to her; the woman may also prefer not to have visitors. There is some evidence that third-day blues are less likely to occur if *bonding between the mother and her baby has been initiated, and if *rooming-in is practised. Third-day blues is in fact a misnomer as the inability to adjust to parenthood, with feelings of inadequacy, tiredness, reduced sexuality, emotional liability, and, in a small proportion of women, severe depression, may persist for weeks or months (see *Depression after childbirth).

Touching

The skin of the human body is a sensitive organ and certain areas arouse sexual excitement. These erogenous areas include the genitals of a male, the breasts and genitals of a female, and the lips of both sexes. Other areas become erogenous for certain people who derive pleasure from touching that particular part of their body or having it touched by their partner. Touching and its more formalized form, body massage, are enjoyable and sensuous experiences, which may be enhanced if scented body-oils or lotions are used and if the pleasuring takes place in a warm, relaxed environment. Touching, caressing, fondling, and massage are often sufficient in themselves for the pleasure they give, or may be used as an erotic prelude to sexual intercourse.

Toxic shock

Toxic shock is a rare condition which occurs most frequently among women who use tampons as a form of *menstrual hygiene. It occurs between 6 and 9 times per year per 100 000 tampon users (or about once every 12 million times a tampon is inserted). It is two and a half times as common in women aged less than 30, and the risk is increased if the woman changes the tampon infrequently.

Toxic shock is due to the release of a toxin from the germ *Staphylococcus aureus*, which may live in the vagina. The toxin is absorbed into the blood and causes a higher fever (38.9°C), vomiting, and diarrhoea; muscle pains; a diffuse sunburn-like red rash; a fall in blood pressure, leading to shock, and one to two weeks later, peeling of skin from the palms of the hands. Treatment is to treat the shock and to give large doses of antibiotics.

Toxic shock can be avoided by changing tampons every 4 to 6 hours in the day, and at night using external pads.

Transsexuality

A transsexual is a person, male or female, who is convinced that he or she is of one sex but has the bodily appearance of the other sex. A female transsexual's feelings and desires are those of a man, but her body is female. This may cause anxiety and misery.

It is not known why certain people believe passionately that they are entombed in the wrong body. There is some evidence that in childhood, transsexuals preferred dressing as a member of the other sex, and for much of the time behaved – discreetly – as a member of the other sex would do.

A transsexual's intense desire is not only to pass as a member of the other sex, but to have the body-shape, and particularly the genital appearance, of the other sex. To achieve this desire demands that a woman receives male hormones, has her breasts, ovaries, and uterus surgically removed, and her genitals reconstructed to give her a form of penis. There is currently much discussion about the ethics of this type of surgery, especially as genital reconstruction is generally of poor quality and the artificial penis of little functional value. In most centres where transsexuality is treated, no person is accepted for surgery until extensive psychological testing has shown that there is no mental illness or personality disorder which could be the basis for the problem. Physical tests are also made to ensure that the person is fit to undergo the hormone treatment and the surgery. The person has to live as a male for at least two years before surgery is contemplated. These conditions are realistic; the controversy arises over surgery. While mastectomy and removal of the ovaries (and uterus) are relatively simple operations, the reconstruction of the genitals is often a surgical disaster. This area of surgery needs considerably more research carried out.

Travel in pregnancy

With the far greater mobility that now exists for holidays or business, many pregnant women may wish to travel by road, rail, air, or sea. Unless a woman has a history of repeated abortions, and provided that she can make the journey in a comfortable way, there are no medical restrictions on travel. Most airlines refuse to carry pregnant passengers after the 32nd week, particularly on long journeys, as they have few facilities for childbirth should the woman unexpectedly start labour.

Trichomonad infection

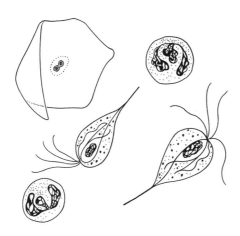

Trichonomonad infections are caused by organisms called trichomonas vaginalis, seen here under the microscope

Trichomonads are microscopic organisms which may infect the vagina causing marked *vaginal discharge (which is sometimes greenish and bubbly) and itching inside the vagina and around its entrance. They are transmitted sexually.

Routine smears taken from women attending family planning clinics or hospital clinics show that between 2 and 10 per cent of sexually active women harbour the organism in their vagina, and in about half of them it causes symptoms.

The diagnosis is made by the doctor examining the discharge under a microscope, or sending a swab for culture. When the diagnosis is made both the woman and her sexual partner should be given treatment. A tablet of metronidazole (Flagyl) or tinidazole (Fasigyn) is taken by mouth three times a day for 7 days; or if the woman prefers, she may take a single dose of 4 tablets. The treatment may cause nausea and a general feeling of being unwell, and occasionally dark urine. Alcohol should be avoided while metronidazole is taken, as the person may experience headache, abdominal discomfort, flushing, and vomiting. Following treatment, vaginal swabs should be repeated, as occasionally a second course of treatment is found to be necessary.

Trophoblastic disease

The common form of this disease is called hydatidiform mole. It occurs because for some reason the embryo or the fetus dies but the placental tissue (trophoblast) continues to grow abnormally. Over a few days or weeks the *placenta is converted into a tumour which fills the uterus with grape-like masses. Trophoblast disease occurs in about one pregnancy in every 2000. The woman usually notices that something is wrong as she starts to bleed, and thinks she is about to abort. She may feel nauseated and when examined may have a raised blood pressure, or a uterus which is larger than expected. The diagnosis is confirmed by *ultrasound. Treatment depends on the woman's age and her desire to have further children. The two choices are to remove the tumour from the uterus using a *suction curette, or to perform a *hysterectomy. As the tumour produces a specific hormone, treatment is followed by taking blood samples at intervals and by measuring the level of the hormone human chorionic gonadotrophin (HCG) in the blood. Normally the level of HCG becomes undetectable about 12 weeks after the hydatidiform mole has been removed from the uterus. If the level does not fall normally, or rises, there is a strong possibility of a trophoblastic malignancy and the woman is offered treatment of *chemotherapy, with a cure rate of over 90 per cent.

Following removal of a hydatidiform mole, the woman should avoid becoming pregnant for at least 12 months, but may use *oral contraceptives if she chooses.

Tubal ligation

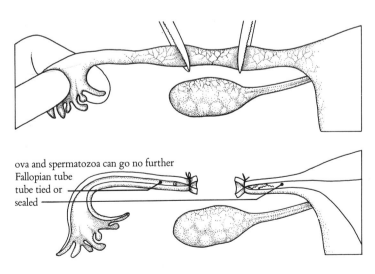

ova and spermatozoa can go no further
Fallopian tube
tube tied or sealed

Increasing numbers of women, when they have completed their family, choose a permanent method of birth control in preference to continuing to use contraceptives. The choices available are for the man to have a *vasectomy or for the woman to have a tubal ligation (sterilization). The choice should be made after the couple have discussed the matter at some length.

Tubal ligation can be performed through a small incision above the pubic hair, or by using a *laparoscope. This instrument, which resembles a hollow, narrow rod, is introduced into the woman's abdominal cavity through a tiny incision below the umbilicus. Another instrument is introduced through a second tiny hole.

The Fallopian tubes are either tied using catgut, or sealed off with a plastic clip kept closed by a small piece of non-corrodable sprung metal which is placed across each tube. These two methods are not usually followed by any problem, but other methods, such as burning part of the tubes, have now been discontinued because they were often associated with problems.

Women who choose tubal ligation should consider the method a permanent one. It is true that if the methods outlined have been used, the operation can be reversed, using microsurgical techniques, but at best only 70 to 75 per cent of women subsequently manage to become pregnant, and the chance of an *ectopic pregnancy occurring is ten times the normal rate.

Turner's syndrome

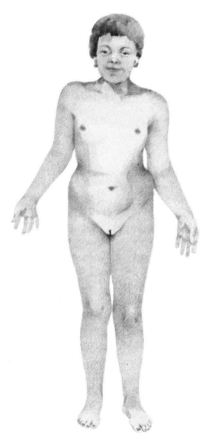

Turner's syndrome in adolescent girls causes short stature, a web neck, no breast development, angled arms and no menstruation

Adolescent girls with Turner's syndrome (gonadal agenesis) fail to have the pre-pubertal spurt of growth, fail to develop breasts, and fail to menstruate. In other words, they fail to show the changes of *puberty. The condition is due to a genetic defect as the child has only one X chromosome instead of the usual two which are essential for the normal development of the ovaries. In consequence, at birth the baby has tiny ovaries which contain no follicles (egg cells) and fail to develop. At puberty, in spite of the normal surge of pituitary hormones, the ovaries are unable to respond and produce *oestrogen (as this is produced in the follicles in normal women). As a result, the breasts remain flat, the genital tract fails to mature, and menstruation fails to occur.

Turner's syndrome is often diagnosed in childhood as the girl may have other signs of the condition, especially a 'webbed neck'. If it is diagnosed, counselling at that time helps the girl (and her family) adjust to the problem. She has to adjust to the fact that she will always be short in height and will never be able to have children. However, she can obtain a feminine figure after the expected age of puberty by being given hormones. The administration of oestrogen in tablet form will lead to the development of her breasts, and her vagina will become mature, so that she can have a normal sexual life, including sexual intercourse.

U

Ultrasound

Ultrasound is a diagnostic medical technique which has been developed in the past twenty-five years. The principle underlying diagnostic ultrasound is that sounds of short wavelengths penetrate tissues and are reflected to a different degree depending on the character of the surface which the sound-wave encounters. The reflected sound-waves can be translated into light dots, which are retained on a cathode tube to produce an image. In the human, ultrasound is used to form a picture of organs and tissues in the body. If a 'real time ultrasound' machine is used, the picture is 'living', and movements and changes in the shape of organs are visualized.

The investigations are safe, as ultrasound does not cause damage to cells in the way that X-rays may, and are painless. In early pregnancy, ultrasound is often used to help in determining if a woman has aborted and, after the 8th week of pregnancy, ultrasound detects the beating of the fetal heart. Later in pregnancy, ultrasound is used to determine the age of the fetus, whether it is growing properly, whether it has a malformation, where it is lying in the uterus, whether there are twins, and to determine the position and limits of the placenta. In gynaecology, ultrasound helps detect an *ectopic pregnancy, to diagnose *trophoblastic disease, and to determine if an *ovarian cyst is present.

Umbilical cord

If the fetus is seen as an astronaut in a space capsule, the umbilicus is the life-line which connects it to its 'life-support' system, the *placenta. The umbilical cord is about the thickness of a finger and contains two arteries (which carry blood to the placenta) and one vein (which carries blood from the placenta). The blood vessels are in a jelly-like substance. The umbilical cord is usually about 50 cm long, but its length can vary from 10 to 120 cm. Despite its length it rarely causes problems for the fetus during labour.

Urinary control

A baby passes urine frequently. If an adult behaved like a baby, all sorts of social problems would arise. To prevent this, an adult learns to prevent urination until the time is appropriate; in other words, the person is continent. Urinary continence or control depends on several factors. The first is that the urethra has an 'inherent tone', which prevents urine passing along it until the pressure in the bladder exceeds that in the urethra. The bladder constantly receives small quantities of urine which trickle down the ureters from the kidneys. The bladder can stretch to accommodate up to 350 ml of urine without the pressure inside it rising. When more than this amount of urine fills the bladder, messages pass from it to the brain and cause the bladder muscle to contract; this raises the pressure in the bladder above that in the urethra so that the person feels uncomfortable and wants to urinate. However, she has learned to suppress the muscle contractions until she is in an appropriate place. When she is, she lets the bladder muscle contract and at the same time increases her abdominal pressure by fixing her diaphragm and pushing downwards. When that happens she passes urine. When a woman is not able to control urination, she is said to suffer from *urinary incontinence, which has a variety of causes.

Urinary incontinence

Urinary incontinence is the name given to the condition when a person is unable to control urination. Women are more prone to the condition than men. Women who have urinary incontinence 'wet' themselves at unexpected and inappropriate times, which can be very embarrassing. There are three types of urinary incontinence. The first is when a woman is constantly wet with urine. This is due to a fistula, a hole between the bladder and the vagina caused by damage during childbirth, after treatment of cancer of the uterus, or sometimes after *hysterectomy. It can be cured by surgery, and is the least common cause of urinary incontinence.

The two other types of urinary incontinence are frequently confused by doctors and may require special investigations. The first type is called *urgency incontinence*. Normally a woman can hold up to 350 ml of urine in her bladder before feeling the urge to urinate. A woman with urgency incontinence experiences an urgent desire to urinate when the bladder is less full, and may wet herself before she can control the desire. She has an *irritable bladder. The treatment of an irritable bladder is not by surgery, but rather re-education of the bladder, 'teaching' it to fill to its capacity.

The other type of urinary incontinence is called *stress incontinence*. In this condition stress, in the form of a cough, or a jump, or during sudden jolting movement, or sometimes even a fit of laughing, leads to a small amount of urine being passed. Stress incontinence is not uncommon in pregnancy (but usually disappears when the baby has been born). It becomes more common as a woman grows older when it can wreck her life, as she becomes very self-conscious and sometimes afraid to go out in case she wets herself. The problem is a weakness of the bladder neck. In stress incontinence the supports of the bladder neck (in the area where it becomes the urethra) weaken and it changes in shape from being like an apple with a stalk to a pear with a stalk. This means that a sudden pressure on the bladder, for example from a cough, pushes urine down and the woman is unable to control the flow before she has wet herself. The treatment of stress incontinence is surgical, which is very successful provided the correct diagnosis has been made.

Urinary tract infection

In the course of their life most women will develop an infection of the urinary tract, at least once. In addition, about 5 per cent of women have a urinary tract infection which causes no symptoms (bacteriuria), but which may flare up, especially in pregnancy. Many obstetricians now have a sample of the woman's urine examined in a laboratory (usually collected when urinating in midstream, hence its term midstream urine, or MSU). Other women develop a frequent need to pass urine and pain on urination which may indicate *cystitis. In a few women the bladder infection tracks up to involve the kidney, causing kidney infection, or pyelonephritis. This is associated with fever, shivering attacks, and backache over the kidney. In all cases a specimen of urine is examined and an appropriate antibiotic prescribed. If an attack recurs, many doctors recommend that an intravenous pyelogram (IVP) be made. This involves injecting a dye into a vein in the arm and taking X-rays which outline the urinary tract.

Uterine growth

During pregnancy, the uterus enlarges to accommodate the growing *fetus. From a pre-pregnancy weight of 50 g it weighs 1000 g by the end of pregnancy. Its growth in the first half of pregnancy is due to the increase in the number of the muscle fibres of

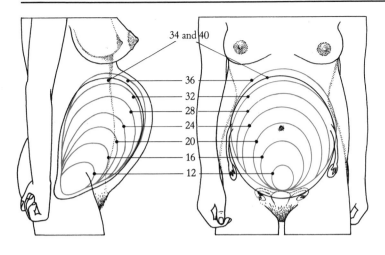

During pregnancy the uterus enlarges at a consistent rate enabling the doctor to palpate the sides of the womb and to assess the length of pregnancy to that point

which it is made, and in the second half of pregnancy its growth is predominantly by an increase in the length of the existing muscle fibres. Uterine growth takes place under the influence of ★oestrogen, which circulates in increasing quantities as pregnancy advances. This permits the cavity of the uterus to expand *in advance* of the size needed to accommodate the fetus, the ★placenta, and the amniotic fluid in which the fetus lives.

One method of estimating how much the pregnancy has advanced is to examine the woman's abdomen to determine the size of the uterus. The method is not very accurate and, if greater accuracy is required for any reason, the doctor may order an ★ultrasound examination. However, in most cases, abdominal palpation is sufficient for the woman and her obstetrician to be sure that the uterus (and also the fetus contained inside it) are growing properly.

Uterine malformations

During the early stages of development of an embryo, the Fallopian tubes, uterus, and vagina develop from two tubes of cells one on each side of the abdominal cavity. The tubes move to approach each other, joining to form the uterus and the upper vagina, and become hollow. If this smooth process fails to occur, the woman may have a single half uterus, an abnormally shaped uterus, two uteri and a single vagina, two uteri and two vaginas, or the vagina may be divided into

two. These conditions are not common but if they occur may cause problems in pregnancy, although most women with a uterine malformation have no trouble. ★Premature birth may occur, or the baby may lie in an abnormal position and may need to be delivered by ★Caesarean section. ★Postpartum haemorrhage is also more likely. In some cases, it is possible that surgery will help to improve the chance of a successful outcome to the pregnancy.

Uterus, contractions

The uterus contracts at intervals throughout pregnancy, but until late pregnancy the contractions are not progressive and are painless. In the last 10 weeks of pregnancy, the painless contractions become more frequent and the woman may feel her uterus become firm for 1 to 2 minutes and then relax. As the time for the birth of the baby approaches the contractions increase in strength, in frequency, and may become painful (★false labour). With these contractions, the uterus contracts as strongly in the lower part as in the upper.

When labour begins, the uterus contracts more strongly in the upper part, and with each contraction the length of each muscle fibre shortens. The effect of this is to pull on the cervix, which opens slowly but progressively in the first stage of labour.

In the early stages of labour it may be difficult to differentiate between the contractions of 'false labour' and true labour. Once the contractions occur every 10 to 15 minutes over 2 hours, the woman is likely to be in true labour. (See also ★Childbirth, labour.)

Vacuum extractor

This instrument, which was originally described 150 years ago, has become popular in the last thirty years, in a modern form, as an alternative to *forceps to deliver a baby. It consists of a flat cap, about 7.5 cm in diameter, which is connected to a vacuum apparatus. The cup is pushed against the head of the baby, and a vacuum created, so it is held against the scalp by the atmospheric pressure. The doctor then pulls on the tubing which connects the cup to the vacuum bottle, and the baby is delivered. The vacuum extractor (or ventouse) is simple to use, and is said to have the advantage that less is introduced into the vagina than when forceps are used. This means that there is less likelihood of damage to the mother's tissues. The instrument causes a circumscribed swelling of the baby's scalp, called a chignon, which takes between 12 and 60 hours to disappear, and about one baby in 7 develops a *cephalhaematoma from the effects of the suction.

Vaginal balls

These are hollow plastic balls measuring 3 cm in diameter which contain movable weights and are attached to each other by a nylon cord. Some women obtain pleasurable vaginal sensations if they place two balls (or more) well inside the vagina. As they walk about, lie down, or sit rocking, the weights move inside the balls imparting a sensual feeling. The balls can also be drawn between the vaginal lips and kept in place by means of a waistband. They are also called Geisha Balls, Benwa Balls, or Thailand Beads.

Vaginal dilators

Vaginal dilators are a series of cylinders made of plastic, glass, or metal which are closed at one end in the shape of a cone. They are graduated in size from the size of a pencil to the size of an erect penis. They are used to help women who suffer from *vaginismus or who have had vaginal surgery to increase the capacity of the vagina. Vaginal dilators are of little value unless used in conjunction with counselling.

Vaginal discharge

During her reproductive years, a woman's vagina is normally kept moist by fluid which seeps between the cells of the vaginal wall. In addition, the surface layer of cells is shed constantly into the vagina, where they react with bacteria which normally live in the vagina to produce a weak lactic acid. The acidity tends to keep the vagina healthy. Under certain conditions such as stress, anxiety, illness, or, sometimes, when the woman is taking the *pill, the normal secretions increase in amount, and form a whitish discharge. This is not irritant but sometimes has an odour. It is called leukorrhoea or the 'whites'. If it is marked, it can be treated with an acid jelly which is inserted into the vagina. A proportion of women, varying from 1 to 15 per cent, nearly all of whom are sexually active, develop vaginal discharges which have a marked odour and cause irritation. Most of these are due to *candida (also called monilia or thrush), *trichomonad infection, or *non-specific vaginitis. A woman who has an irritating vaginal discharge should consult a doctor.

Occasionally, the 'vaginal' discharge is caused by infection of the cervix, the 'glands' of which produce secretions. This may be due to *gonorrhoea and swabs have to be taken from the cervix and the urethra.

Vaginal hygiene

The vagina is normally clean, and its walls lie close together so that it is not an open cavity until something is introduced into it. Its cells produce a mild acid which helps keep it clean. When a woman passes urine some may enter the vagina, but this does not make the vagina dirty, as urine is sterile. Nor does semen as it too is sterile.

One way in which the vagina can be contaminated is if any of the bowel contents enter it, for faeces are not clean: they are heavily contaminated. For this reason a woman should wipe her anus (back passage) after passing a motion, from the front towards the back to avoid transferring bowel contents into the entrance to her vagina.

Vaginal odour

The vagina is kept moist by fluid seeping between the cells which make up its wall. In the cavity of the vagina, the fluid and the cells which are shed from the upper layer of its wall are acted upon by bacteria to produce a mild acid. This acts as a defence against infection. The vaginal secretions have a slightly fishy smell, which may concern some women who believe that the smell can be detected by others. If a woman is concerned, she should wash the hair around the entrance to her vagina regularly and should avoid wearing tight pantihose. Douching does not help and vaginal deodorants should be avoided as it is possible they may cause an allergic vaginitis (inflammation).

Vaginal spermicides

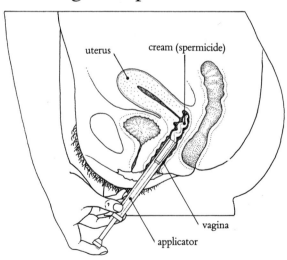

uterus — cream (spermicide)

vagina

applicator

Vaginal spermicides are creams, jellies, foams, and pessaries containing a chemical which immobilizes and kills spermatozoa ejaculated in the vagina. Used alone they are rather ineffective in preventing pregnancy, and between 25 and 35 per cent of women who use this method become pregnant in each year of use. Vaginal spermicides have an important role when used in conjunction with a vaginal diaphragm or if the man uses a ★condom. Used in this way they reduce the likelihood of an unwanted pregnancy. (See also ★Contraception, barrier methods.)

Vaginal spermicides can be supplied in various forms. The illustration shows cream being inserted into the vagina

Varicose veins

Varicose veins are being diagnosed in an increasing number of people and they affect between 10 and 20 per cent of adults, the frequency increasing with age. Usually the leg veins are affected but some women develop varicose veins of the vulva. The increased frequency may be due partly to dietary habits, notably the use of refined flour, leading to less bulky motions and increased difficulty in emptying the bowels. Varicose veins are also more likely to occur in certain families, so that there may be a genetic cause. The condition occurs when the valves along the course of the vein become defective and permit the blood to distend the vein. The result may merely be ugly, but it may also cause aching legs and some discomfort on standing. Treatment is to wear supportive stockings or to have the varicose veins dealt with surgically. This can be done either by injecting drugs into segments of the relevant vein in order to obliterate it, or by having an operation which 'strips' the vein out of the leg.

Vasectomy

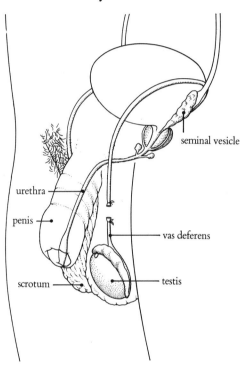

urethra

penis

scrotum

seminal vesicle

vas deferens

testis

Vasectomy is an operation in which the man's vas deferens – the tube which carries spermatozoa from his testes to his penis – is divided. The vas can be felt if the man's scrotum is palpated gently, at the level where it joins his body, by putting a thumb in front and an index finger behind and rolling the folds of skin between them. The vas is felt as a cordlike structure. Under local anaesthesia (or a general anaesthetic, if the man prefers) a small incision is made in the skin of the scrotum, and the vas is identified and cut; the operation takes about 15 minutes. Sexual intercourse can resume as soon as the couple wish, but some form of contraception must be used until the man has ejaculated about twelve times. This is because he has to ejaculate the spermatozoa which are stored in his prostate gland. After this he is sterile. The operation has no side-effects; it does not reduce the man's sexual desire, arousal, or pleasure and it is easier to perform than a *tubal ligation on a woman.

Vasectomy – male sterilization is a simple operation in which the vas deferens is blocked so that sperm cannot pass through to the penis, instead they dissolve and are absorbed

Venous thrombosis

One woman in a hundred is affected during pregnancy or after childbirth by a clot in a leg vein (venous thrombosis). Venous thrombosis occurs more frequently among those women who are overweight, who are over the age of 35, who smoke, and who take the *pill. Older women needing major operations are at greater risk of developing a clot in a leg vein or in a vein in the pelvis. If the vein affected is a deep vein, the clot may become detached and travel in the blood to the lungs where it may cause a pulmonary embolus. Because of this danger, women who develop clots in deep veins, or who require major surgery after the age of 60, are often given injections of an anti-clotting drug called heparin, to reduce the chance of an embolus occurring.

Version of the fetus

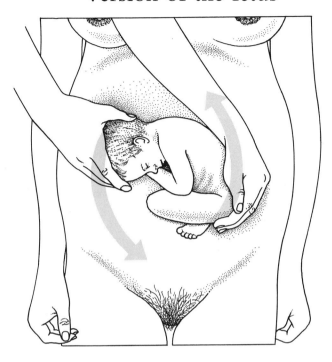

By the 35th week of pregnancy over 90 per cent of fetuses have settled to lie in the uterus head downwards. The other 10 per cent lie either with the breech presenting or transversely (see ★Fetal positions in pregnancy). If a doctor finds a breech presentation when he examines a woman who is 34 weeks pregnant, he may suggest that he 'turns' the baby so that it becomes head down. The reason is that birth is safer for a baby presenting cephalically (head down). The manoeuvre is done gently, without anaesthesia, and is abandoned if the baby does not turn easily. Occasionally a doctor will perform a version in labour. Usually this is done if a second twin is lying in an unfavourable position in the uterus. The doctor introduces his hand into the uterus through the vagina, and 'brings down a leg', converting the presentation of the baby into a breech.

Vibrator

Vibrators are made in the shape of a disc or as a plastic cylinder which resembles an erect penis in shape and size. The apparatus contains a small electric motor which is powered by a battery or from the mains supply. When switched on the vibrator produces a rhythmical, gentle side-to-side movement. Vibrators create a warm, pleasant sensation when pressed against the skin, and are used for body massage. If a vibrator is applied to the clitoral area or the penis it leads to sexual arousal and to orgasm. Some women and men obtain a more intense orgasm using a vibrator than from masturbation or sexual intercourse. Vibrators are useful in several areas: they help women become aware of their orgasmic potential and are used to treat failure to reach orgasm; in the absence of a partner, a vibrator may be preferred to digital stimulation of the clitoral area; they can also be made use of during ★sexual pleasuring. After use the vibrator should be washed thoroughly in soap and water and dried well before being put away.

Virilism

A few women undergo body changes which make them less feminine and more masculine; this is known as virilism. The woman's clitoris enlarges, her breasts diminish in size, she grows hair on her face, typical male baldness develops, her voice deepens, and her menstrual periods cease. In most cases, the condition develops because a tumour of the ovary or of the adrenal gland, or because over-activity of the adrenal gland, releases an increased amount of the male hormone testosterone into the blood. Occasionally, virilism occurs because the woman is given injections or tablets of testosterone to treat a lack of sexual arousal or because she has *premenstrual tension. Investigations by hormone analysis and body scanning have to be made so that the appropriate treatment can be given. If the condition is caused by a tumour of the ovary or the adrenal gland, the virilism will be reversed when the tumour is removed.

Vitamins

A healthy person who eats a nutritious, prudent *diet does not require additional vitamins taken in tablet or capsule form. A few people in the industrialized nations will benefit from vitamin supplements, especially elderly people who eat a poor diet, but most vitamins consumed in large (and increasing) quantities by many women pass unchanged through their body to join the sewage, and help the bacteria multiply. Pregnant women are frequently prescribed vitamins, or believe that they should take additional tablets. There is no evidence that a healthy woman living in a developed country requires any vitamin supplements, except for some Asian women living in Britain who require extra amounts of vitamin D, because of their diet and life-style.

Vitamins are also taken to prevent or cure disease, though again there is no real evidence in most cases that the vitamin helps. Careful studies show that large amounts of vitamin C neither prevent cancer nor colds (although the severity of the cold may possibly be reduced). Vitamin B-complex pills (containing thiamin or pyridoxine) do not relieve premenstrual breast pain or even *premenstrual tension more effectively than sugar pills. Vitamin E has not been shown to benefit the heart, the skin, sexual potency or to prevent ageing; it remains a vitamin 'in search of a disease'. Vitamin K, which prevents haemorrhage in newborn babies, is an exception. An injection is usually given at birth to tide the baby over until he forms his own source by the end of the first week of its life.

Vitamins are beneficial and can aid in preventing disease among poor people in the developing nations of the Third World. Vitamin A given to infants and children will prevent blindness; vitamin B will prevent beriberi and pellagra from developing; vitamin D will prevent rickets.

Vulva, itchy

Itchiness of the external genitals is a not uncommon symptom, which can be distressing to a woman and requires careful investigation. About half of the affected women will be found to have *candida or *trichomonad infections.

A few women have a generalized skin condition, and a few have diabetes. When vaginal 'hygienic' douches were popular, a few women developed an allergy, and today the wearing of synthetic pantihose may cause vulval itchiness. In about one-third of patients who have an itchy vulva no cause is found after investigation. It has been suggested that in younger women, anxiety, sexual frustration, or depression may be causes; while in women after the *menopause, the lower amounts of *oestrogen circulating in the blood leads to a thinning (atrophy) of the skin of the area, which causes an itch. Itchiness is an allergic reaction which is caused by the release of histamine-like substances, in response to a challenge, either physical or mental. (See also *Itching, perianal.)

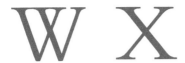

W X

Weight, 'desirable'

Life insurance companies have access to a large amount of information in which the weight, height, and age of people are related to their chance of developing certain diseases, or of those diseases becoming more incapacitating. A person whose weight is in the 'desirable' range is least likely to be affected by the diseases. The information relating to a desirable weight can be given in a table or a chart, and is usually shown as a range: a woman whose weight for her height and age lies within a range between 20 per cent below and 20 per cent above the 'desirable' or 'ideal' weight is said to have a 'normal' weight.

Another method of discovering if your weight is within the normal range uses a calculation devised over a hundred years ago. It is this: divide your weight in kilograms (W) by the square of your height in metres (H^2). The formula W/H^2 gives an index, as set out below:

Emaciated	less than 15
Underweight	15 to 17.9
Normal weight	18 to 24.9
Overweight	25 to 29.9
Obese	30 to 40
Severely obese	More than 40

Weight gain in pregnancy

During the 40 weeks of pregnancy, well-nourished women gain an average of 12.5 kg. In the first 20 weeks about 3.5 kg is gained; in the second 20 weeks the weight gained increases to about 0.5 kg a week or 9 kg over the whole period. The weight gain in pregnancy is made up of several components, as itemized in the table.

It is believed that the fat stores of 3.5 kg are an evolutionary device to make sure that the woman has a large reserve of energy to enable her to provide breast milk for her baby. The additional energy released from the fat store is equal to 30000 kcals (125.4 MJ). As the daily energy cost of producing milk is about 500 kcals (2.1 MJ) a day, the energy that is provided from the fat store is of particular value.

Distribution of weight gained	20 weeks	40 weeks
Fetus	300 g	3500 g
Placenta	200 g	600 g
Uterus/breasts	800 g	2200 g
Blood (increase in volume)	400 g	1200 g
Fat	1400 g	3500 g
Fluid (in tissues)	400 g	2600 g
	3500 g	12500 g

Withdrawal

On a world-wide basis, withdrawal (coitus interruptus) is a common method of fertility control. The man withdraws his penis from the woman's vagina immediately before orgasm so that he ejaculates outside the vagina. There are two main problems with coitus interruptus as an efficient method of contraception: first, the man has to be sufficiently motivated and athletic to withdraw before he ejaculates; and second, a small amount of ejaculate, containing spermatozoa, may seep out of the penis before withdrawal.

Coitus interruptus is potentially disadvantageous for the sexual needs of a woman as the man may ignore her desire to reach orgasm and she may also lose the pleasure of feeling him reach orgasm, with his penis contained in her vagina. However, it need not necessarily disadvantage a woman sexually, if she can express her sexual needs to her partner and he is able to respond sufficiently to these.

Worms

Intestinal parasites (worms) affect large numbers of people, particularly children, throughout the world. In the developed nations, the most common worms are threadworms and roundworms, but tapeworms also occur. Roundworms and tapeworms cause few symptoms unless the infestation is heavy; but threadworms may cause an intensive itch around the anus and around the vulva in women. This is because the female worm emerges from the gut (usually at night) to lay her eggs around the anus, and her movements are responsible for the itch. If a strip of adhesive tape is applied to the skin around the anus in the morning and taken to the doctor for examination, the eggs of the worm can be seen, and treatment will be given. (See also *Itching, perianal.)

Wrinkles

As the skin ages it becomes stretched and weathered, so that it appears wrinkled. In many cultures, wrinkles were a sign of knowledge and maturity and older people were respected. In our youth-oriented society, wrinkles are an indication that a person has passed the peak of attractiveness.

Several things increase the likelihood of wrinkles. These are heredity; exposure during adolescence and young adulthood to sun and sea-wind; marked changes in weight; and possibly heavy cigarette-smoking.

It has recently been suggested that facial massage and exercises may increase, not decrease, wrinkles, but the truth of this has not yet been confirmed.

The only way wrinkles can be eliminated is by covering them up with make-up, or by having a face-lift. A face-lift eliminates wrinkles – for a time, but the ageing process goes on inexorably and the newly smooth face begins to wrinkle again. Creams containing *oestrogen or vitamin E are often recommended, but are not effective. Oestrogen enables the skin cells to retain water temporarily so that the wrinkles appear less obvious, but to maintain the effect, the hormone would have to be used each day. As this causes oestrogen to be absorbed into the blood, it is possible that this may cause unpleasant side effects in the woman. (See also *Skin 'foods'.)

X-rays in pregnancy

In the 1930s, an X-ray examination of a pregnant woman's pelvis to determine its size was considered an essential prenatal investigation. In addition to this, X-rays were used to diagnose twins, breech presentation, some fetal abnormalities to determine the maturity of the fetus, and to confirm the diagnosis of death of the fetus in the uterus.

It is now known that X-rays should be used with care in pregnancy so that the potential danger of radiation to the fetus is avoided. In many cases, *ultrasound can be used in place of X-rays, and gives more accurate information. However, in some instances, X-rays may help the obstetrician in making a diagnosis, particularly if ultrasound is not readily available. If a modern machine is used and the radiologist is careful, there will be no harm to either the mother or the fetus.